A NOTE FROM THE AUTHOR

I have discovered in the last few years that the subject of health has become increasingly important to me. Of the books I have done about health, this book on diagnostic tests best reflects my passion. Here's why:

Most of us know more about our cars than our bodies.

Perhaps the only way to achieve better health, to reduce health costs, is by individual permission to embrace preventive medicine, to head off disease, to be one step ahead of illness through the multitude of tests described herein. The right test at the right time should be no different than getting your oil changed or your chassis lubed on a regular basis.

We should take better control of the laboratory that is our body.

If you care about someone...

If your livelihood depends on someone...

Consider buying this book as a gift of love and learning.

RSW

A NOTE FROM THE AUTHOR

I have discovered in the last few years that the subject of health has become increasingly important to me. Of the books I have done about health, this book on diagnostic tests best reflects my passion. Here's why:

Most of us know more about our cars than our bodies.

Perhaps the only way to achieve better health, to reduce health costs, is by individual permission to embrace preventive medicine, to head off disease, to be one step ahead of illness through the multitude of tests described herein. The right test at the right time should be no different than getting your oil changed or your chassis lubed on a regular basis.

We should take better control of the laboratory that is our body.

If you care about someone...

If your livelihood depends on someone...

Consider buying this book as a gift of love and learning.

RSW

DIAGNOSTIC TESTS FOR MEN

Meet Dr. Seemore. He'll be dispensing additional advice and interesting facts alongside the descriptions of the tests, the procedures involved, and the results of the tests in this section of the book.

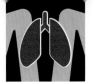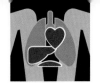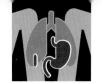

INTRODUCTION

You probably have this book in your hands because your doctor has recommended that you have a diagnostic test, and you want to know more about what you will experience. **Many men will skip this introduction and open the page for the test they are going to take.** That's fine. But if you would like to know a little more about medical diagnostic tests for men in general, or about the suggested tests for men at different ages, read on.

Some words of reassurance

The great majority of screening tests recommended for men by doctors are not cause for alarm or anxiety. They are routine preventive measures to be certain that your body is healthy and functioning normally. **These tests are important because the majority of diseases—even the most serious ones—can be cured or controlled when discovered in early stages.** A few of the routine tests are uncomfortable, embarrassing, or as painful as the sting of a hypodermic needle. Most are minimally invasive and painless. The best news is that the vast majority of all preventive tests reveal that the patient is healthy and problem-free.

An overview of medical testing for men

Ironically enough, as a statistical generality, **doctors are better equipped to test men than they are to test women.** Just a few years ago, two-thirds of all clinical trial participants were men, which means that there is a huge body of male-specific medical data. There are distinct biological differences between women's and men's organs and organ systems, and certain diseases affect one sex but not the other, or affect the two sexes differently. But the fact is that men really hate going to the doctor, even for tests—which could be life-threatening, particularly as men grow older. Only four out of every eleven adults visiting a doctor are male. Despite the fact that, statistically, men live seven years less than women, women are 1.5 times more likely to consult a doctor than men. Men need to visit their doctors for regular checkups and exams—more frequently as they grow older. In specific, doctors have become more vigilant in testing men for cardiovascular disease, high blood pressure, throat and lung cancer, and bladder cancer. Heart disease develops ten years earlier in men than in women—**men have more than three times as many heart**

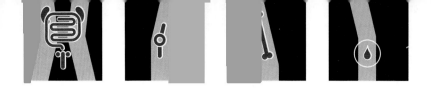

attacks as women—424,000 every year in the 45-64 age group. Although 93% of lung cancer is directly linked to tobacco use, 27% of all American men over 18 continue to smoke, and men are twice as likely as women to have throat/mouth or lung cancers. Men who drink more than six drinks a week have double the risk of fatal illness that moderate drinkers or non-drinkers have. African-American men have a 33% higher death rate from cardiovascular disease than white males. Osteoporosis, long considered a woman's problem, actually affects 20% of older men. Men are prone to higher rates of visual loss and hearing impairment than women after age 45.

Issues in testing for men
The largest single problem in medical testing is fear—not of the tests, but of the results. Unhappily, fewer than 40% of all men have a regular physical exam. Even fewer have the necessary screening for colorectal cancer, despite an 85% cure rate for cases detected in early stages. For most men the motivation is the ease of mind provided by good reports or the early detection of problems. Despite careful laboratory procedures and skilled diagnostic analysts, test results can be incorrect. Some estimates suggest that there is a 50% chance of error in the normal panel of blood tests. In most cases in which an abnormality is detected, a doctor will order the same test again or another test for verification.

An important issue is the interpretation of test results. If your doctor diagnoses a condition based on tests, you should discuss the medical evidence found with him or her and feel comfortable asking about the possibility of error. If you are not completely confident in the answers you receive, do not hesitate to seek a second opinion. Particularly in the diagnosis of life-threatening diseases, the majority of doctors will welcome consultation with a colleague. Most HMOs and insurance companies will approve payment for a second opinion in serious cases. Be certain to ask about the advantages and alternatives to any treatment.

Finally, it's up to you
Your best assurance of thorough, competent testing is your own cooperation and communication with doctors and technicians. You should initiate a dialogue about the testing and ask questions about the procedures. **Read the information in this book and be empowered. Take responsibility for your own health.**

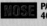

HEART PAGE 44

Electrocardiogram
(EKG or ECG)
page 46

Chest X-ray
page 46

Echocardiogram
page 47

Angiography
page 48

Nuclear heart scan
page 48

Electron beam
computed
tomography
page 49

Cholesterol,
triglycerides
page 49

Apolipo-
proteins
page 50

Heart enzyme,
CPK, CK,
SGOT, LDH
page 50

Vitamin B1
page 50

Hematocrit
page 50

Anti-
myocardial
antibodies
page 51

LUNGS PAGE 52

Arterial
blood gases
page 54

Carboxy-
hemoglobin
page 54

Pulmonary
function test
page 54

Bronchogram
page 55

Bronchoscopy
page 55

Mediastinoscopy
page 56

Sputum culture
page 56

Thoracentesis
page 56

Lung scan
page 57

LIVER PAGE 58

Endoscopic
retrograde
cholangio-
pancreatography
page 60

Abdominal
ultrasound
page 61

Computed
tomography of
the biliary tract
and liver
page 61

Percutaneous
liver biopsy
page 61

Mono spot
blood test
page 62

Alanine
Aminotransferase
blood test
page 62

Alpha-feto-
protein blood test
page 63

Alkaline
phosphatase
blood test
page 63

Bilirubin
blood test
page 63

Protein, albumin,
serum protein,
globulin and
serum
electrophoresis
blood tests
page 63

Hepatitis
blood test
page 64

Ammonia level
blood and
urine test
page 64

more

5

UPPER GI
PAGE 80

Fecal occult
blood test
page 82

Gastrin
blood test
page 82

Upper GI series or
barium swallow
page 82

Esophagogastro-
duodenoscopy
(EGD) or
Gastroscopy
or Upper GI
Endoscopy
page 83

Gastric analysis
page 83

Helicobacter
pylori tests
page 84

KIDNEYS
PAGE 66

Electrolytes
page 68

Magnesium
page 68

Osmoality
page 68

Phosphorus
page 69

Sodium
page 69

BUN
(blood urea
nitrogen),
Creatinine,
Creatinine
clearance
page 69

Urinalysis
page 69

Urine amino
acid screen
page 70

Urine culture
page 70

24 hour urine
(steriods,
calcium,
protein &
estrogen)
page 70

Abdominal
x-ray
page 71

Cystography,
cystoureth-
rogram
page 71

Pyelogram
page 71

Renal
angiogram
page 71

Cytoscopy
page 72

Cystometry
page 72

Renin assay,
plasma
page 72

Renogram,
renal scan
page 73

GALLBLADDER & PANCREAS
PAGE 74

Endoscopic
retrograde
cholangio-
pancreatography
page 60
(Liver)

Oral
cholecystogram
page 76

Percutaneus
transhepatic
cholangiography
page 76

Amylase
page 77

C-peptide
page 77

Glucose
page 77

Hemoglobin AIC
(glycohemoglobin)
page 78

Ketones
page 78

Lipase
page 79

Sweat test
page 79

LOWER GI
PAGE 86

Routine stool
lab tests
(occult
blood, stool
and rectal
cultures)
page 88

Proctosigmoid-
oscopy or
sigmoidoscopy
page 88

Colonoscopy
page 89

Barium enema or
air contrast enema
page 89

CT colonoscopy
page 90

Laparoscopy
page 90

Carcino-embryonic
antigen blood
test (CEA)
page 90

Rectal digital exam
page 91

As medical technology advances, new diagnostic tests become available to consumers, often before they become accepted procedures by the medical profession. Recent developments include the combination of sophisticated computer analysis and various imaging methods to provide fast, noninvasive, three-dimensional views inside all parts of a body–all for a price. For example, a full body scan using electron-beam computed tomography costs approximately $500 to $725. A PET scan which screens your body by function rather than by structure can run as much as $2,000 to $3,000. Low dose CT scans which are often used to study a specific organ, say the lungs, are a bargain at $200 to $300. Critics argue that these tests engender unnecessary expense, cause undue worry to healthy people, and have no measurable benefit for the majority of people tested. Few insurance companies will pay for these scans as preventive tests. However, if you are willing to pay, there is no better way to visualize what is happening inside your body.

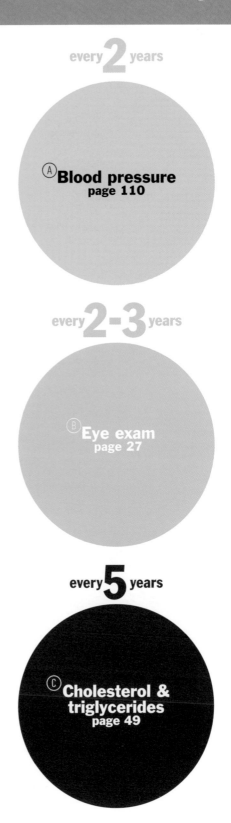

every **2** years

(A) **Blood pressure**
page 110

every **2-3** years

(B) **Eye exam**
page 27

every **5** years

(C) **Cholesterol & triglycerides**
page 49

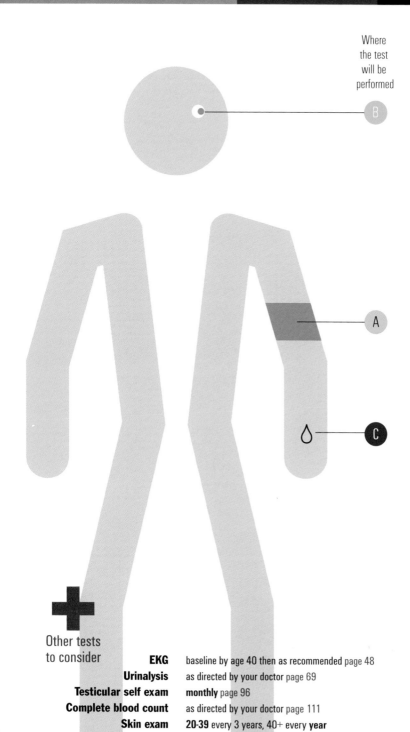

Where
the test
will be
performed

B

A

C

Other tests
to consider

EKG	baseline by age 40 then as recommended page 48	
Urinalysis	as directed by your doctor page 69	
Testicular self exam	monthly page 96	
Complete blood count	as directed by your doctor page 111	
Skin exam	**20-39** every 3 years, 40+ every **year**	
Sexually transmitted disease screen	as directed by your doctor	

What tests should you take

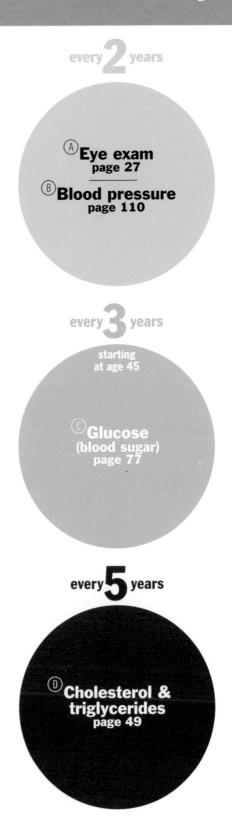

every **2** years

Ⓐ**Eye exam**
page 27

Ⓑ**Blood pressure**
page 110

every **3** years

starting
at age 45

Ⓒ**Glucose**
(blood sugar)
page 77

every **5** years

Ⓓ**Cholesterol &
triglycerides**
page 49

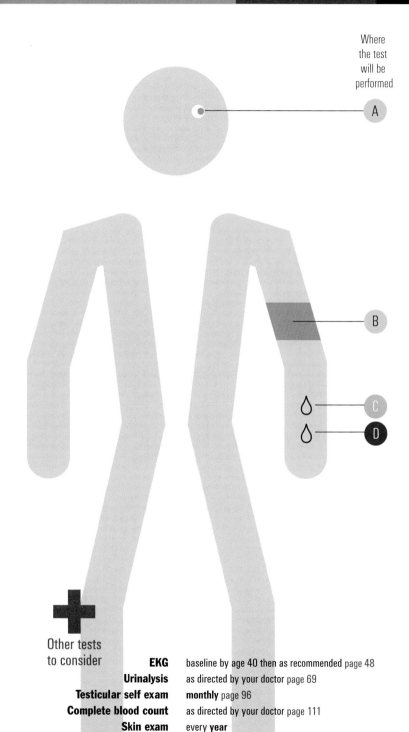

Where
the test
will be
performed

A

B

C

D

Other tests
to consider

EKG	baseline by age 40 then as recommended page 48
Urinalysis	as directed by your doctor page 69
Testicular self exam	monthly page 96
Complete blood count	as directed by your doctor page 111
Skin exam	every year
Sexually transmitted disease screen	as directed by your doctor

What tests should you take

every year

Ⓐ **Fecal occult blood**
page 88

Ⓑ **Prostate specific antigen**
page 94

every 2 years

Ⓒ **Eye exam**
page 27

Ⓓ **Blood pressure**
page 110

every 3 years

Ⓔ **Glucose** (blood sugar)
page 77

every 3-5 years

Ⓕ **Colon exam**
pages 88–89

Sigmoidoscopy, Colonoscopy or Colon X-ray

(Colonoscopy is most comprehensive but may not be covered by insurance.)

every 5 years

Ⓖ **Cholesterol & triglycerides**
page 49

Ⓗ **Digital rectal exam**
page 91

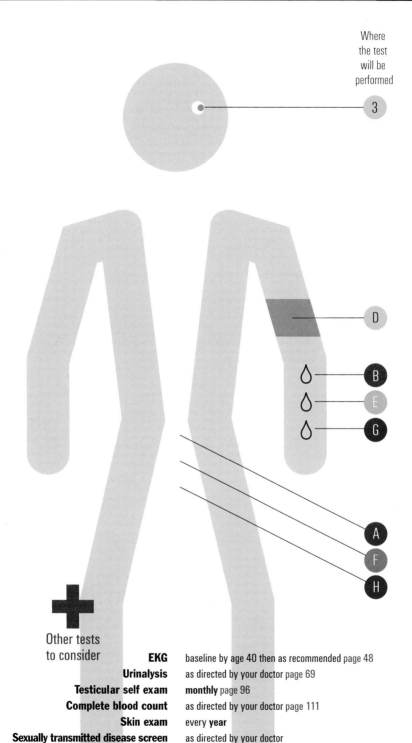

Where
the test
will be
performed

3

D

B

E

G

A

F

H

Other tests
to consider

EKG	baseline by age 40 then as recommended page 48
Urinalysis	as directed by your doctor page 69
Testicular self exam	monthly page 96
Complete blood count	as directed by your doctor page 111
Skin exam	every **year**
Sexually transmitted disease screen	as directed by your doctor

What tests should you take

every year

Ⓐ **Eye exam**
page 27

Ⓑ **Fecal occult blood**
page 88

Ⓒ **Prostate specific antigen**
page 94

every 2 years

Ⓓ **Blood pressure**
page 110

every 3 years

Ⓔ **Glucose**
(blood sugar)
page 77

every 3-5 years

Ⓕ **Colon exam**
pages 88–89

Sigmoidoscopy, Colonoscopy or Colon X-ray

(Colonoscopy is most comprehensive but may not be covered by insurance.)

every 5 years

Ⓖ **Cholesterol & triglycerides**
page 49

Ⓗ **Digital rectal exam**
page 91

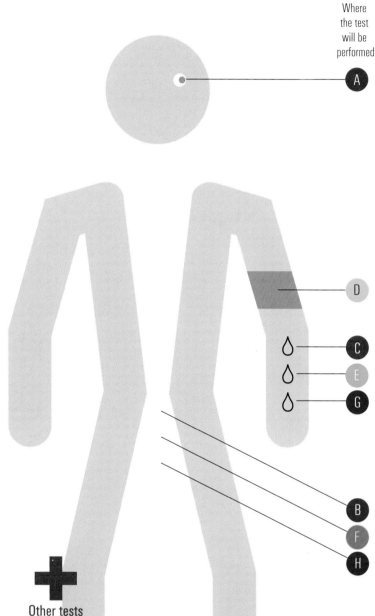

Where
the test
will be
performed

A

D

C

E

G

B

F

H

Other tests
to consider

EKG	baseline by age 40 then as recommended page 48	
Urinalysis	as directed by your doctor page 69	
Testicular self exam	monthly page 96	
Complete blood count	as directed by your doctor page 111	
Skin exam	every year	
Sexually transmitted disease screen	as directed by your doctor	

What tests should you take

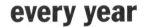

every year

(A) **Eye exam**
page 27

(B) **Fecal occult blood**
page 88

(C) **Prostate specific antigen**
page 94

every 2 years

(D) **Blood pressure**
page 110

every 3 years

(E) **Glucose**
(blood sugar)
page 77

every 3-5 years

(F) **Colon exam**
pages 88–89

Sigmoidoscopy,
Colonoscopy
or Colon X-ray
(Colonoscopy is most
comprehensive but may not be
covered by insurance.)

every 5 years

(G) **Cholesterol & triglycerides**
page 49

(H) **Digital rectal exam**
page 91

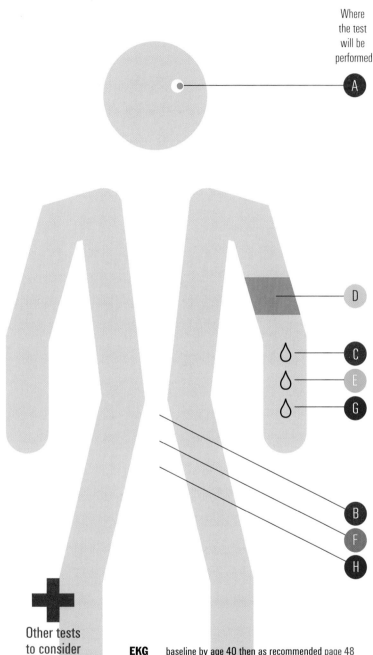

Where
the test
will be
performed

A

D

C

E

G

B

F

H

Other tests
to consider

EKG	baseline by age 40 then as recommended page 48
Urinalysis	as directed by your doctor page 69
Testicular self exam	monthly page 96
Complete blood count	as directed by your doctor page 111
Skin exam	every year
Sexually transmitted disease screen	as directed by your doctor

17

18

At birth, the human brain weighs about three-quarters of a pound, and certain areas of the newborn forebrain show no electrical activity at all until the age of seven or eight months. The average **adult** brain weighs approximately three pounds. There is no correlation between normal variations in human brain size and intelligence.

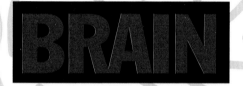

BRAIN

The brain is the major organ of the nervous system, and the primary
computer of the human body. It is composed of more than one hundred billion nerve cells, each of which is connected to thousands of others, which make it far more complex than any mere computer— and more sensitive.

Brain disorders are treated by a neurologist, who specializes in problems of the nervous system. These problems may have either physical or behavioral manifestations. Many brain-related disorders such as mental retardation, are evident at birth, though some may develop during life. Other disorders include stroke, brain tumor, blood vessel abnormalities (aneurysms), epilepsy/seizures, migraines headaches, and other neurological diseases.

Cancers of the brain are among the most common brain diseases. They affect not only the brain itself, but also the part of the body regulated by the region of the brain impaired by the tumor. This unique aspect of the brain—its function as the control center of the systems of the body—makes treatment a sensitive issue.

From middle age onward, the most important threat to the brain is impaired blood supply

to one or more brain regions, which causes the death of irreplaceable brain cells. If an artery within the brain becomes blocked or ruptures, causing hemorrhage, the result is called a *stroke*. Risk factors for stroke include age, high blood pressure, arteriosclerosis (plaque buildup in arteries), diabetes, and smoking. Stroke kills approximately 144,000 people in the United States annually, 40% of whom are men.

Alzheimer's disease (AD) is the most common cause of dementia in older people. The disease usually begins after age 65, and the risk of AD goes up with age. It affects about 3 percent of men and women aged 65 to 74, and nearly half of those over age 85 may have the disease. Nevertheless, **Alzheimer's is not a normal characteristic of old age.**

6 QUESTIONS TO ASK YOUR DOCTOR

? If I think I have a problem with my brain, what should I do right away?

? What is the best test to diagnose my particular symptoms?

? Do I have any conditions that would make a particular test a bad idea?

? Are there any restrictions on my diet or activities before the test?

? Does the clinic or hospital require a patient consent form in order to take this test?

? How will I feel after the test?

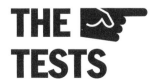

THE TESTS

CHEMICAL MESSAGE CENTERS

Major glands in the body's endocrine (hormone-producing) system

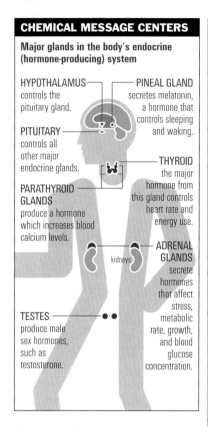

HYPOTHALAMUS
controls the pituitary gland.

PITUITARY
controls all other major endocrine glands.

PARATHYROID GLANDS
produce a hormone which increases blood calcium levels.

TESTES
produce male sex hormones, such as testosterone.

PINEAL GLAND
secretes melatonin, a hormone that controls sleeping and waking.

THYROID
the major hormone from this gland controls heart rate and energy use.

kidneys

ADRENAL GLANDS
secrete hormones that affect stress, metabolic rate, growth, and blood glucose concentration.

Hormone Testing

The presence of hormones in the blood and urine is regulated in part by the brain and its subsidiary organs. Too much or too little of various hormones can be signs of brain malfunction. Hormones in the blood may be functionally important, and hormones in the urine may signify disease.

Procedure

Blood and urine—collected in the usual manner—can both be tested for hormones moving through the body. Blood or urine samples may require fasting or may need to be taken early in the morning, depending on the hormone. In certain cases, 24 hour urine testing may be required.

Results

High or low levels of cortisol in the blood indicate malfunction of the pituitary or adrenal glands. Often this suggests a tumor in one of these glands.

Testosterone, an important male hormone, has a normal range of production. Anything outside of this range indicates malfunction of the pituitary gland. Tumors can cause this malfunction, as can a malfunctioning thyroid (See **THROAT** pages 41-42).

Pituitary hormones regulate much of the body, particularly the reproductive functions. Malfunctions in these organs lead to testing these hormones in the blood. Again, tumors or a malfunctioning thyroid may be the cause.

Spinal Tap or Lumbar Puncture

In this test, fluid which flows around the brain and spine is withdrawn for analysis.

Procedure

An area in the lower back or back of the neck is anesthetized and sterilized. A needle in then inserted into the lower back between two vertebrae to withdraw the fluid that bathes the brain and spinal cord. This fluid flows up and down the spinal column and around the brain, as well. Proper insertion may require several tries and can be painful.

Results

The cerebrospinal fluid is a leading indicator of problems in the brain and spine. It is usually clear, and the presence of almost any type of cells in the fluid can indicate infection or leakage from the brain. The fluid's pressure may be taken as well.

Cerebrospinal fluid may be tested for:

Alzheimer's Disease

The presence of Amyloid Beta Protein can be an indication of Alzheimer's and other dementias.

Bleeding

Detection of red blood cells may indicate bleeding from an aneurysm.

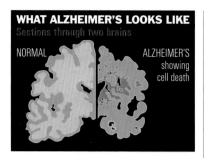

WHAT ALZHEIMER'S LOOKS LIKE
Sections through two brains

NORMAL

ALZHEIMER'S
showing
cell death

Many tests and a large overview are often needed to diagnose Alzheimer's. A.D. is a clinical diagnosis, not a laboratory test diagnosis.

An estimated 4 million people in the U.S. suffer from Alzheimer's Disease. Alzheimer's begins with forgetfulness and the inability to do simple tasks, such as math problems. These difficulties build with time, and the ability to think clearly diminishes as well. Speaking, understanding, reading, writing, and caring for oneself all fade slowly as well.

Meningitis
The fluid may be examined under a microscope or cultured to test for meningitis, an infection of the meniges (the membranes that cover the brain and spinal cord.)

Multiple Sclerosis
If certain proteins are found, MS may be diagnosed.

Computerized Axial Tomography (CAT or CT Scan)
This type of scan can be useful anywhere on the body, but particularly on the brain. It provides sharp, two and three dimensional images of the brain and can be used to localize tumors, clots or other brain abnormalities.

Procedure
In the case of the brain CAT scan, the patient lies on a table which moves into the scanner. The patient must lie motionless while the scanner takes pictures, for up to an hour.

Sometimes an iodine contrast dye is injected, which can help obtain clearer pictures. Although rare in the newer, fast scanners, and scanners that are "open" on the sides, some patients experience claustrophobia and may require a sedative.

Results
Symptoms such as headaches, dizziness, seizures, extremity weakness or numbness usually lead to this test. Possible causes of these problems that this test can detect are brain tumors, evidence of a stroke, or treatable causes of dementia.

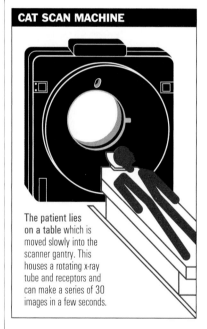

CAT SCAN MACHINE

The patient lies on a table which is moved slowly into the scanner gantry. This houses a rotating x-ray tube and receptors and can make a series of 30 images in a few seconds.

Doppler Ultrasound
This type of ultrasound is particularly capable of detecting motion, such as blood flow in veins and arteries. It may show arterial narrowing or blockages.

Procedure
As with all ultrasounds, a hand-held probe is passed over the area of interest and the sound waves are converted to a picture. In this case, large vessel blood flow to the brain can be observed.

more tests

Results

The technician or doctor can see and report immediately any abnormalities that are observed. Clots, arterial plaques or obstructions that cause strokes can be detected, along with blood flow patterns in the brain which can show evidence of dead tissue in parts of the brain.

Electroencephalography (EEG, Brain Wave Test)

This painless test measures the electrical impulses produced by the brain, which usually appear in a normal pattern. In order to measure electrical activity in the brain, electrodes wired to a machine are applied to the scalp, and readings are taken. Abnormal brain wave patterns can assist the doctor in diagnosing brain tumors, stroke, blood clots, epilepsy and seizures.

Procedure

The patient lies down, and up to 30 electrodes are adhered to the scalp with conductive gel. These are attached to a machine which graphs brain activity over time. The patient lies still, may be shown bright lights, put to sleep with a sedative, or asked to breathe heavily as the machine takes readings. This test lasts up to an hour, at which time the electrodes are removed. The electricity flows from the brain to the machine; there is no risk that it may be reversed.

Results

Abnormal patterns in the EEG waves can indicate brain tumors in a specific area, evidence of a stroke, blood clot or epilepsy, but the most common use is to detect seizures or brain malfunction. The test is also used to establish whether a person is brain-dead.

A variation of this test, called an Evoked Potential Study, provides external stimulus to the brain during the EEG. The brain is tested to see how quickly it responds. Any signifi-

cant time lapse can indicate brain damage or damage to the optic nerve or nerves to the ears.

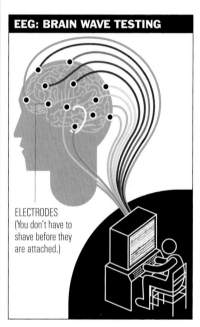

EEG: BRAIN WAVE TESTING

ELECTRODES
(You don't have to shave before they are attached.)

Electromyography

This test examines the function of nerves in the body. In particular, it investigates the electrical pathways between the brain and the muscles it controls.

Procedure

The patient must lie on a table, and electrodes are adhered with gel to the nerve pathway or muscles to be tested. These are attached to a meter which measures electrical current. As the patient tenses and relaxes certain muscles, the electrical output is measured. Under any circumstances, this test is uncomfortable. However, current may be passed between the electrodes as well to stimulate the muscles, which briefly may produce a burning sensation.

Results

The results of this test appear in three ways: on a graph similar to an EEG graph, on a monitor, and as popping noises over a loudspeaker as the

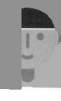

nerves fire. The doctor can interpret this collection of data, detecting nerve and brain disease which damages muscle function. Diseases such as multiple sclerosis, myopathy, diabetes, polio, and ALS (Lou Gehrig's Disease) may be diagnosed. This test is usually ordered with signs of muscle weakness or pain.

Magnetic Resonance Imaging (MRI)

This test can be performed on most parts of the body and provides excellent magnetic images, but is particularly useful for the brain. When the results are viewed, tumors, aneurysms, multiple sclerosis and infection are clearly visible.

Procedure

As with all MRIs, the patient lies on the MRI table, which slides into the machine. The patient lies still as the imager thumps and moves around for 30 to 90 minutes. In some cases, just before the test begins, a safe contrast dye may be injected in a vein to provide greater clarity. Although perfectly safe, the MRI imager is disconcertingly more noisy than a CAT scan, and some patients may feel claustrophobic and require a sedative or an "open" scanner.

CHOICES AMONG BRAIN TESTS: CAT VS. MRI VS. PET

The CAT scan, although it involves slightly more radiation than a normal X-ray, can produce clear images of the brain in less than half an hour. The MRI is exceptionally safe. It involves no radiation and usually no contrast dyes. It can produce images of the brain, blood vessels and some detail of the skull. However, it is an especially expensive test. PET scans produce unusually precise images of brain activity based on metabolic activity. This sophisticated technique allows doctors to "see" brain activity in real time as thoughts are developing. Unfortunately, the cost of PET scans is prohibitive, because the radioisotopes must be produced in a cyclotron.

Results

The images produced are examined by a doctor, who can see the entire area examined. Tumors, aneurysms, blood clots, blood flow, and hemorrhages will be clear to a trained specialist.

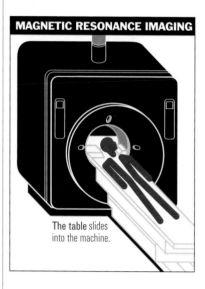

MAGNETIC RESONANCE IMAGING

The table slides into the machine.

Octreotide Scan

This nuclear test is used to investigate the status of known tumors, primarily brain tumors.

Procedure

A radioactive substance (sometimes called a radionuclide) is injected into a vein, from which it spreads through the body. This substance is absorbed in greater concentrations by different types of tissue, so that the tissues can be distinguished by a sensitive type of machine that reads levels of radiation, called a gamma camera. This gamma camera (which translates the x-ray-like gamma rays into images) can take pictures of the entire body and show different tissues in clear contrast. Unlike the dyes that are used in cardiac catheterization or coronary angiography, radionuclides carry virtually no risk of toxicity or allergic reaction.

Results

The pictures track the radioactive

substance through the body. If the radionuclide has attached to tumors, these should be apparent in the pictures. Tumors can be found and their progress monitored with this test.

Positron Emission Tomography Scan (PET)

This imaging test combines techniques from two common forms of tests: the nuclear scan and biochemical assessment.

Procedure

This test begins with the inhalation or injection of a radioactive element through an IV. Often, a second IV line is required to obtain serial blood samples periodically during the test. The radioactive element, as it decays in the body, emits nuclear energy when metabolized. The patient lies on a table which slides, like a CAT scan, into a large scanning device. The energy can then be measured by scanners. The speed at which the nuclear energy is released allows doctors to observe the metabolism of the patient. The energy emitted can be traced to specific organs, and images can be made based on the speed and location of this energy. This test may sound frightening, but it is safe, nontoxic, and subject to the mild discomfort or claustrophobia of any scan test. Also, recent use of caffeine, alcohol, or tobacco—or brain-influencing drugs such as tranquilizers—may affect test results.

Results

PET traces the distribution pattern of the radioactive substances injected, and translates this information into color pictures. Like the CAT or MRI scans, the PET is used to search for unusual masses in the body. It detects them by the speed at which they attract and metabolize the nuclear element in the body. Tumors, as well as evidence of heart attacks and strokes, can be seen. Single Photon

Emission Computed Tomography (SPECT) is a similar type of test, which uses slightly different technology. SPECT scanning recognizes abnormal cells by their abnormal metabolism, not by their abnormal appearance.

LEFT BRAIN, RIGHT BRAIN

The brain is divided into left and right hemispheres that specialize in different forms of activity. The hemispheres are connected by the **corpus callosum**, a bridge of a hundred million nerve fibers (**shown in red**). Differences in hemispheric specialization develop in individuals between birth and age 12.

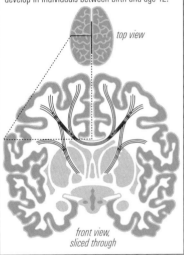

top view

front view, sliced through

SYMPTOMS OF STROKE

The most common stroke symptoms, too often ignored, include

- dizziness
- sudden loss of consciousness
- confusion
- double vision or sudden deterioration in vision
- slurring of speech
- partial paralysis or numbness.

Treatment within three hours of a stroke can make the difference between permanent disability or death and normal function. The more quickly you react to stroke symptoms in yourself or others, the more likely you may be able to minimize permanent damage.

TOP WAYS TO AVOID A STROKE

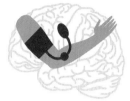

Control your **blood pressure**
with appropriate medication.

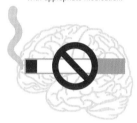

Don't smoke

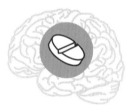

Take one **aspirin** per day
(in consultation with your doctor).

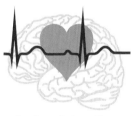

Treat **heart rhythm** problems
with vigilance.

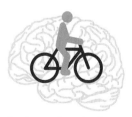

Practice a regular routine of proper
diet and **exercise**.

For further information

Alzheimer's Association
Suite 1000
919 North Michigan Ave.
Chicago, IL 60611-1676
800-272-3900
www.alz.org

National Headache Foundation
Dept. PF
5252 N. Western Ave.
Chicago, IL 60625
778-878-7715

American Council for Headache
Education
800-255-ACHE
www.cs.uu.ne/wais/html/na-bng/
alt.support.headaches.migraine

National Stroke Association
96 Inverness Drive East
Suite I
Englewood, CO 80112-5112
1-800-STROKES (1-800-787-6537)
www.stroke.org

National Institute of Neurological
Disorders and Stroke
Information Office
P.O. Box 5801
Bethesda, MD 20824
1-800-352-9424

Neurosciences on the Internet
www.neuroguide.com

The Parkinson's Web
www.pdweb.mgh.harvard.edu

Dana BrainWeb
www.dana.org/brainweb

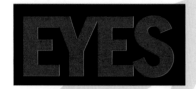

The normal human eye blinks about 25 times each minute. Eyestrain from working on the computer or reading too long may be the result of insufficient blinking.

The poet who said that "the eyes are the windows of the soul" was only half right. They are windows into the workings of the body, too.

All ophthalmologists and optometrists study ways in which the eyes reflect the health of the entire system. An examination of the arteries and veins visible in the back of the eye can reveal signs of high blood pressure, arteriosclerosis, brain disease, diabetes, and other problems throughout the body. **Diabetes is often linked to vision problems at all ages,** and is the leading cause of blindness in adults between the ages of 20 and 74. It accounts for over 8,000 new cases of blindness each year. Other vision problems may be evident from birth. Babies born prematurely are often vision-impaired, and some full term babies need glasses in infancy. The availability of laser surgery provides the opportunity for permanent vision correction

6 TOP QUESTIONS TO ASK YOUR EYE CARE PROFESSIONAL ABOUT YOUR GENERAL HEALTH

- Do the arteries look healthy and normal?
- Is there any suggestion of high blood pressure?
- Is there any evidence of developing diabetes?
- Are my eyes in good health for my age?
- Can you observe normal optic reflexes?
- Are any blood clots visible?

and is becoming increasingly common. These vision surgeries, used to treat nearsightedness, farsightedness and astigmatism, are expensive but usually accurate one-time procedures — however, laser surgery can have complications and requires careful consultation with your eye care professional before deciding to proceed.

Light travels from the optic nerve to the back of the brain at 300 miles per hour.

Most tests for the eyes are simple, painless, and noninvasive.

A few of the more sophisticated tests for macular degeneration or optic nerve damage may require hospital-based x-ray or scanning technology, but most eye diagnostics are conducted by eye care professionals during regular office visits.

During a routine checkup, the patient goes to a private room, and drops are often put into the patient's eyes. These drops dilate the pupils, opening them wider so that the inner workings of the eye and the back, called the retina, are easier to observe. As a result, these drops may blur vision and make the eye sensitive to light. Driving, reading and any activity in bright sunlight should be avoided for several hours after the drops are administered. Patients may want to call ahead to ask if someone else should drive home. Different drops are also used to numb the eyes, so that surface tests can be performed without discomfort; these do not cause distortion of vision.

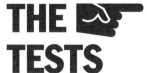

THE TESTS

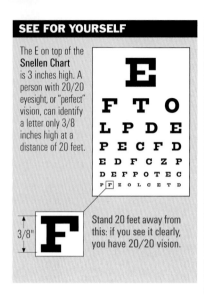

The E on top of the **Snellen Chart** is 3 inches high. A person with 20/20 eyesight, or "perfect" vision, can identify a letter only 3/8 inches high at a distance of 20 feet.

3/8"

Stand 20 feet away from this: if you see it clearly, you have 20/20 vision.

Visual Acuity

This common test measures how well the eye can see. The Snellen Eye Chart, first used in 1862, still hangs on most physicians' walls, with its large E on top. This test is performed at nearly every general physical, as well as during every visit to an eye care professional.

Procedure

The chart, with its rows of rapidly shrinking letters, is set 20 feet from the patient, who must then read down the chart until the letters are no longer clear. The test is done one eye at a time, and first done without glasses, then with them, if the patient wears them. A chart with other symbols may be used for preschoolers and patients who are not familiar with the Western alphabet.

In addition to distance vision, a Jaeger card is used to test near vision. This card works just like its larger cousin, with rows of letters which decrease in size. The card is placed at a set distance from the patient, who then reads until the letters are no longer clear. The Jaeger card can be used to determine a prescription for reading glasses or bifocals.

Results

Visual acuity is expressed as a fraction, the top portion of which is always 20, indicating the 20-foot distance from the patient to the Snellen chart. The bottom portion of the fraction compares the patient's eyesight against the norm. Someone with 20/60 vision sees at 20 feet what those with perfect vision can see at 60 feet, and cannot discern the smaller letters on the chart that are clear to someone with 20/20 vision. This simple test is used (often in conjunction with phorometry—see below) to determine accuracy of vision. If reading the chart proves very difficult, it might indicate a more serious problem, such as glaucoma or cataracts.

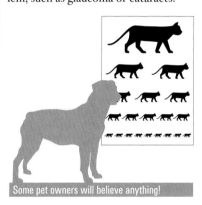

Some pet owners will believe anything!

Phorometry

A phoropter is an instrument with many different lenses that test the eyes' ability to focus. Phorometry involves looking at the Snellen Chart (*see above*) through these goggles, which place adjustable lenses in front of the eye.

Procedure

The phoropter is lowered over the face and different lenses are placed between the eye and the chart. The patient is asked to judge which lens makes the letters appear clearer, and the lenses are increasingly fine-tuned as the test goes on. The patient is asked to judge the clarity of vision in each eye for distance and close-up vision.

GETTING THE RIGHT LENSES

The phoropter

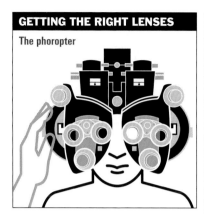

Results
The goal of this test is to determine the strength of glasses or contact lenses to be prescribed.

Visual Field Test (Perimetry)
This test measures the sensitivity of your retina to light across different areas of the visual field.

Procedure
The patient rests his head in a chin rest, facing a bowl shaped instrument. A series of lights go on and off and the patient is asked to respond to what is seen.

Results
The absence or reduction of sensitivity in one or more areas may indicate one or more disorders, including glaucoma.

Color Defectiveness Determination
True color blindness, in which everything appears black and white, is relatively rare. Color defectiveness or color deficiency is far more common. This test measures the ability to discern differences among various colors.

Procedure
The test involves looking at a series of slides which have color patterns on them. The patient will be asked to identify what is on the slide.

Results
Within the color patterns are numbers and letters which are obvious to normal eyes, but not to those that are color defective. Several types of color defectiveness exist which make two different colors appear the same. For example, red-green color-blind people cannot distinguish these two colors.

COLOR BLINDNESS

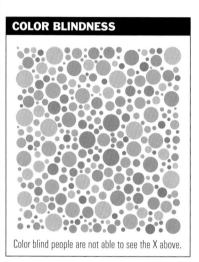

Color blind people are not able to see the X above.

About ten times more men than women are color blind. The most common color deficiency is red/green. Inability to detect the color blue is very rare.

Muscle Integrity Evaluation
This test evaluates the health and function of the muscles which control eye movement.

Procedure
The doctor or technician directs the patient to perform simple motions with the eye—back and forth, up and down. These eye movements are observed by the doctor.

Results
If there is any problem moving the eye, or a discrepancy between the response of one eye and the response

more tests ▶

of the other, it could indicate muscle or nerve damage or deterioration.

The definition of legal blindness in the US is determined in two ways. First, if no better than 20/200 corrected vision can be attained in a person's better eye, he or she is considered legally blind. Second, if a person's tunnel vision is so far advanced that the visual field is restricted to 20 degrees or less, they also are legally blind.

Glaucoma is the second leading cause of irreversible blindness in the US, and the leading cause among African-Americans. The incidence of glaucoma is four to six times higher in blacks than in whites, and it becomes more prevalent with age. Among whites, glaucoma is present in 0.5-1.5% of persons under age 65 and 2-4% of those over 75. Among blacks, 1.2% of those between the ages of 40 and 49 and 11.3% of those over 80 have glaucoma. Prevalence of glaucoma is increased in patients with diabetes mellitus, myopia, and a family history of glaucoma. Of the various forms of glaucoma, primary open-angle glaucoma (POAG) is the most common in the US (80-90% of cases), and is estimated to be responsible for impaired vision in 1.6 million Americans and blindness in 150,000.

Dry Eye Test (Schirmer Tear Test)

This test assesses the functioning of the lacrimal glands in the eye, and measures the quantity of tearing.

Procedure

After the patient is seated comfortably in an examining chair, he is asked to look up and a sterile strip of filter paper is gently inserted under each of the lower eyelids. After a period of time, usually five minutes, the strips are removed from the patient's eyes and the length of the moistened area on the filter paper is measured in millimeters.

Results

A Schirmer test strip should show at least 15 mm of moisture after five min-

utes. Because tear production decreases with age, 10 mm would still be within the normal range for patients over the age of forty. The problem of "dry eyes" is normally associated with aging, although rarely may result from systemic diseases. Up to 15% of the patients taking the Schirmer test have false-positive or false-negative results. Because the test is quick and simple, it is usually repeated to compare results in question.

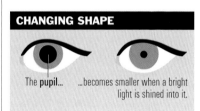

CHANGING SHAPE

The pupil... ...becomes smaller when a bright light is shined into it.

Pupillary Reflex Response

This test measures how fast the pupil closes when confronted by a bright light.

Procedure

Whenever the eye is exposed to bright light, the pupil is supposed to become smaller. A bright light, shined by the doctor or technician into the eye, should trigger this response.

Results

The closure of the pupil in the presence of bright light is a reflex. When light shines into the eye, any abnormality in the response can be an indication of nerve damage, damage to the cornea, or damage to the iris, which controls the pupil.

Keratoconus, a progressive thinning of the cornea, affects one in every 2,000 Americans, and is most prevalent in teenagers and adults in their 20s. It can be detected during routine eye exams and treated with contact lenses in 90% of the cases. Advanced cases may require corneal transplants.

Floaters, which appear to the patient as spots that "float" across the field of vision, can also be a sign of deterioration of the retina, although more often they are normal visual defects that inhibit vision only slightly. New floaters may be associated with a retinal tear or detachment.

Slit Lamp Exam (Biomicroscopy)

The slit lamp is a device which examines the front of the eye. A doctor can see the surface, cornea, and lens up close in order to determine that they are in healthy condition.

Procedure

The eyes are sometimes dilated with drops, and the patient is instructed to sit forward and rest the chin on the slit lamp apparatus. The doctor then moves the lamp around to look into the eye while the patient looks straight ahead. One variation of this test involves introducing fluorescein dye into the eye, either by drops or on a paper strip which is touched to the eye. This dye spreads across the surface of the eye, and stains any cuts, tears, or foreign bodies, making them easy to observe.

Results

The eye should appear normal and healthy. The doctor can see scratches on the surface of the eye, as well as damage to the eyelids, cornea, or lens of the eye. The doctor can also detect infections, inflammations and the presence of foreign objects lodged in the eyeball.

Intraocular Pressure Determination (Tonometry)

This test measures the internal pressure of the eye, and should be performed with each eye examination.

Procedure

After anesthetic drops are put in the eye, the front of the eyeball is touched gently with a pen-like tube, the tip of which measures pressure. This is slightly unnerving but not uncomfortable or painful. A variation on this procedure is the "air puff" tonometry, which requires no direct contact, but can also accurately measure pressure.

Results

High pressure can be an indicator of something wrong within the eye, although not all abnormal pressure indicates glaucoma. Many patients with high pressure (perhaps more than 70%) will never develop vision problems due to glaucoma. However, this test is extremely important as a preventive measure, and early detection can save loss of vision.

More and more, evidence says that tonometry is not as closely related to glaucoma as once thought. High-risk patients may want to seek the newer technology of the Hillelberg Retinal Tomograph.

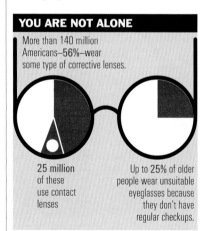

YOU ARE NOT ALONE

More than 140 million Americans—56%—wear some type of corrective lenses.

25 million of these use contact lenses

Up to 25% of older people wear unsuitable eyeglasses because they don't have regular checkups.

Retinal Examination (Direct Ophthalmoscopy or Fundoscopy)

This test is a way for the doctor to examine the inside and rear of the eye. The retina is the only place in the body where blood flow can be noninvasively observed.

more tests

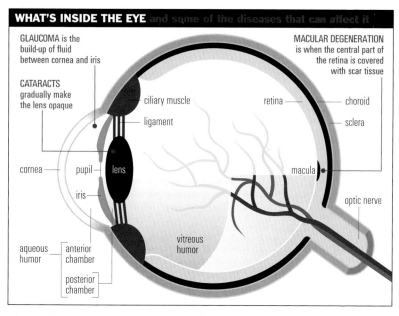

WHAT'S INSIDE THE EYE and some of the diseases that can affect it

GLAUCOMA is the build-up of fluid between cornea and iris

MACULAR DEGENERATION is when the central part of the retina is covered with scar tissue

CATARACTS gradually make the lens opaque

ciliary muscle

ligament

retina

choroid

sclera

cornea

pupil

lens

iris

macula

optic nerve

aqueous humor

anterior chamber

posterior chamber

vitreous humor

Procedure

Using a small instrument with a small beam light source and magnifying lens (the ophthalmoscope), the doctor peers into the eyes and asks the patient to fix on a point, while the doctor moves the light source for examination. The bright light, especially if the eyes have been dilated, can be uncomfortable to look at.

Results

This test allows the doctor to get an idea of the general health of the body, and may reveal whether a patient has high blood pressure or diabetes. The doctor also can see the retina at the back of the eye and determine whether there is any damage to it. "Floaters" become visible, as does any retinal detachment or the beginning signs of macular degeneration. Although rare, blood clots from a stroke, tumors, or fluid attributed to meningitis infections may be visible as well.

Another version of this test, called Binocular Indirect Ophthalmoscopy, uses brighter light and dilation drops. The doctor uses a lamp which can be attached to the head, or another light source and hand-held magnifying lenses through which light can be shone. By focusing and directing brighter light, more of the eye can be seen, and in greater detail.

Orbital Computerized Tomography Scan

This specialized form of CAT scan (the orbit is a medical term for the eye socket area) may be required for a clearer view of eye anatomy, to determine the cause of abnormal protrusions of the eyeball, or to diagnose brain-related disorders or circulatory disorders. Though standard x-rays of the orbit are often used for similar purposes, the CAT scan gives a more three-dimensional view of the eye and its surrounding structures.

Procedure

As with other CAT scans, the goal is to obtain extremely detailed x-rays. All hair clips, jewelry or other objects are removed. The patient lies flat on a table, and the head is placed in a stabilized, cushioned area which slides into the scanner, a large-doughnut shaped instrument. To ensure clear images, the patient must lie completely still. The scanner moves around the head, clicking and taking pictures which can then be interpreted by a computer and converted into images. Although the test takes half an hour, the patient may become uncomfortable lying stationary on a hard table for this length of time. Often, after the initial scan is completed, a dye is injected into the arm and the scan is repeated (*see also Fluorescein Angiography*).

Results

The scan is looking for brain-related disorders, such as blood clots, nerve damage or tumors, which can manifest themselves in vision problems. This scan may also help doctors to assess eye damage caused by thyroid disease or bony orbit fractures in trauma injuries. If abnormalities such as bumps develop within the eye, the scan can help identify their cause. These may be foreign objects, infections, blood clots or tumors.

Sight deteriorates naturally with time and degenerative disorders become more prevalent with age. The three most common vision problems affecting people over 50 are presbyopia (a natural aspect of aging that blurs the near vision, correctable with reading glasses), glaucoma (a build-up of pressure in the eye that, untreated, can result in blindness), and cataracts (protein build-up causing a clouding of the lenses that surgeons repair by replacing the lens). Periodic check-ups will routinely include tests for these diseases. Their causes are largely unknown, although genetics and overall health contribute to most.

Eye Ultrasonography

The ultrasound can differentiate among tissues of different densities and is thus useful for close observation of the eye, and to test for abnormalities.

Procedure

The patient is seated in a large chair,

and anesthetic drops are placed in each eye. After the room is darkened, an ultrasound transducer, a pen-like device, is touched to the eyeball in several places. Sound waves transported through the eye and back to the device are recorded as images on a screen. This may be slightly uncomfortable, but the time to "sound" both eyes is less than ten minutes.

How to give your eyes a quick rest in the midst of prolonged reading or computer work: Look out a window and/or focus on objects at a distance. Tilt your head back, chin to the ceiling, and roll your head from side-to-side gently with your eyes open. Raise your eyebrows, keep your head still, and look up.

Results

This test can distinguish tumors and other abnormalities from normal tissue in the eye. Ultrasound can also locate and identify any suspected foreign object which might be lodged in the eye

Fluorescein Angiography

This photo process identifies many problems, including retinal infections or other infections deep in the eye. Damage to the blood flow to and within the eye as well as macular degeneration are also detectable using this test. (see angiography in the terms section)

Procedure

Although this test is one of the most serious eye diagnostics, it can cause only slight discomfort. After the eyes have been dilated, fluorescein dye is injected into an arm vein, causing the vessels of the retina to turn bright orange almost immediately. The injection is moderately painful, like a pin prick, and the dye can sting or cause the patient to feel faint. Allergic reactions are possible as well,

more tests

so the patient must disclose all allergies to the doctor. With the patient's chin resting against the camera, bright flash pictures are taken of the eye every few seconds, for about a minute. Because the eyes have been dilated, this brightness will probably be uncomfortable. Afterwards the patient's urine will be colored orange for several days as the dye passes out of the body.

THE AMSLER GRID

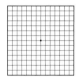

As seen by someone with normal vision

As seen by someone with macular degeneration

Macular Degeneration is a disease which has received growing interest from the medical profession in the past few years. The macula, an area in the middle of the retina, starts to lose its light sensitivity, causing the vision to blur. Sometimes this is due to blood vessels growing into the area, which can be treated with laser surgery. Aside from this procedure which may slow its spread, however, there is no cure. It typically occurs in both eyes, but symptoms usually appear in one eye first. Although women are at greater risk for macular degeneration than men, smoking, high cholesterol, and genetic predisposition may also contribute to the disease, which is usually brought on by age.

Macular degeneration affects about 5% of people over 65, but the risk is about 30% for those over 75. In 1997, $75 million was allocated by the National Institutes of Health specifically to study the disease.

Results

This test produces images of the inside and back of the eye, particularly the veins, which are illuminated by the dye. Blood flow in the eye and the retina can be observed. Circulatory disorders as well as retinal detachment or degeneration is visible. This test is often used to assess and monitor diabetic retinopathy.

The prevalence of cataract increases with age. In persons, aged 55-64 years, one study found 33% of the respondents with early cataract and 6% with late cataract. In persons over 75 years, these figures were 37% and 52%. The frequency of visually significant cataract is lower in men than in women. "Early cataracts" are those that cause no symptoms. "Late cataracts" cause symptoms or have functional significance.

Electroretinogram (ERG)

This sophisticated test observes the functioning of rods, cones, and the optic nerve.

Procedure

After numbing and dilation (or widening) of the pupils, electrodes are placed on the head of the reclining patient. Contact lenses wired to electrodes are inserted in the eyes. The electrodes measure eye movement and response to a series of light flashes and patterns shown in a darkened room. Because the eyelids are held open, this test is disconcerting and uncomfortable. However, the eyes stay moist with drops administered by the doctor or technicians.

Results

By measuring response to light, this test diagnoses nerve damage or other malfunctioning within the eye. Deviations from normal response can indicate such damage.

A-Scan (Ocular Biometry)

If a patient has been diagnosed with cataracts and surgery is necessary to replace the lens, this test is performed.

Ophthalmologists are physicians who spend two to four additional years studying the eyes after they graduate from both college and medical school. They can write prescriptions for eyeglasses, contacts, and drugs, as well as perform necessary tests, procedures, and surgeries.

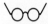

Optometrists are Doctors of Optometry who examine, diagnose, treat and manage diseases and disorders of the visual system. They are empowered to write prescriptions for eyeglasses and contact lenses, low vision aids, visual therapy, and a limited range of drugs to treat eye diseases. They may also perform certain surgical procedures.

Opticians are trained according to state regulations to fabricate, fit and adjust eyeglasses and contact lenses. They are authorized to instruct patients in the proper use of eyeglasses and contact lenses. However, in order to provide eyeglasses or contact lenses for a client, they must first have a prescription from an ophthalmologist or optometrist.

Procedure
The eyes are dilated, and a light shined into the eye measures the power of the current lens.

Results
Using computer technology, the shape, thickness and power of the eye's natural lens is determined, so that a plastic replica with the same focusing properties can be made and placed in the eye during cataract surgery.

Corneal Topography and Corneal Pachymetry
These tests are used to determine the patient's eligibility for laser vision correction and to diagnose corneal disease.

Procedure
During a pre-surgery exam, sophisticated equipment is used to take measurements of the cornea's thickness and map the curvature of the eye's surface.

Results
If topography reveals an irregular-shaped cornea or pachymetry finds a too-thin cornea, you may be rejected for laser surgery.

A few tests not listed here may be performed on the eye. Most of these are non-location specific tests which are widely diagnostic. Information on these tests can be found elsewhere in the book or in the terms section. These tests include: MRI, PET and X-ray,

For Further Information

National Eye Institute
2020 Vision Place
Bethesda, MD 20892-3655
(301) 496-5248
www.nei.nih.gov

American Optometric Association
243 Lindbergh Boulevard
St. Louis, MO 63141
(314) 991-4100
www.aoanet.org

American Academy of
Ophthalmology
655 Beach Street
Box 7424
San Francisco, CA 94109-7424
(415) 561-8500
www.eyenet.org

EAR, NOSE & THROAT

The Ear, Nose and Throat (ENT) specialty is called Otorhinolaryngology—oto for ear; rhino for nose; and the larynx is the voice box area of the throat. An otorhinolaryngologist spends fours years studying this specialty after graduation from both college and medical school.

These areas offer opportunities for doctors to obtain indications of general health in addition to information about a specific organ.

As with other senses, many disorders and diseases of the ears and nose are age-related, and should be tested for more frequently as we age. Some of the common complaints in these areas include hearing loss, vertigo (dizziness), and tinnitus (ringing in the ears). Sinus problems, congestion, post-nasal drip and difficulty with swallowing are noted often as well. The exposure of the ears, nose, and throat to the outside world makes them quite susceptible to infection. There is a modern class of antibiotics called aminogly-cosides, which include drugs such as gentamycin and tobramycin, that may cause damage to both the hearing and balance functions of the inner ear, as well as to the kidney. Surprisingly, the most common ear toxin is aspirin: large doses cause tinnitus or ringing.

THE TOP 6 SIGNS OF HEARING LOSS

- Mistaking words in conversation or missing notes at a concert.
- Not realizing that the doorbell or phone has been ringing.
- Suspecting friends and relatives of mumbling intentionally.
- Withdrawal from social situations if frustrated with hearing.
- Constant ringing or hissing in the background.
- Some sounds are very loud and annoying.

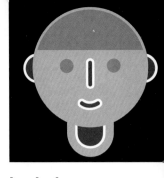

The most common form of hearing impairment in people between adolescence and age fifty, especially for the estimated 5 million Americans with occupational exposure to hazardous noise levels, is noise-induced hearing loss. Hearing can be damaged by one intense, loud noise, or by constant exposure, such as that in a factory. Noises above 90 decibels, such as a jet plane, a rock concert, or a jackhammer, are all risks for hearing damage. The ear can often adjust to loud noises, but unexpected noise can cause irreparable damage. Only rarely, though, does an eardrum actually rupture.

The human sense of smell usually functions in tandem with the sense of taste. However, the nose is approximately 10,000 times more sensitive than the tongue. When your nose is blocked, you lose nearly 90% of the taste sensations.

The thyroid gland, located at the front of the throat, produces the hormones which control the body's metabolism and energy use. The thyroid is an endocrine gland which produces hormones that are carried throughout the body by the blood stream. Thyroid dysfunction affects 1% to 4% of adults in the United States. Thyroid diseases, such as hypothyroidism (the thyroid does not produce enough hormones, making the body sluggish), hyperthyroidism (the opposite of hypothyroidism, making the body agitated), and thyroid cancer, are less common among men than women. Goiter, an enlarged thyroid, is often visible as a swelling of the neck. The thyroid is such a source of medical difficulty for some people that they may be referred to an endocrinologist for diagnosis and treatment. Tests of the thyroid are usually ordered when symptoms of its malfunction are observed elsewhere in the body.

THE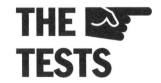
TESTS

EARS

Audiometry (Hearing Test)
Audiometry tests a patient's range of hearing.

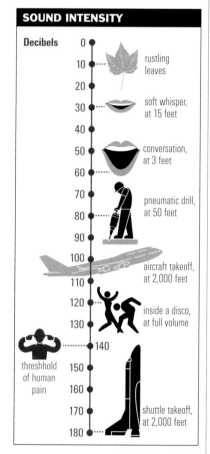

SOUND INTENSITY

Decibels	
0	
10	rustling leaves
20	
30	soft whisper, at 15 feet
40	
50	conversation, at 3 feet
60	
70	pneumatic drill, at 50 feet
80	
90	
100	aircraft takeoff, at 2,000 feet
110	
120	inside a disco, at full volume
130	
140	
150	threshhold of human pain
160	
170	shuttle takeoff, at 2,000 feet
180	

Procedure
In a soundproof room, the patient is usually asked to listen to sounds with and without headphones. A technician pipes tones of different pitches into speakers in the room or into the headphones. The patient is asked to indicate when a tone is heard, and whether it is heard in the right or left ear. By varying the pitch of the tone, the hearing range or the nature and extent of hearing loss can be determined.

Results
The test looks for hearing damage due to trauma or deterioration over time. A hearing aid may be recommended if hearing is found to be damaged.

Prolonged ringing of the ears or pain from sound are indications of severe hearing damage. As a person goes deaf, the high tones generally go first, then speech becomes both difficult to understand and construct. Eventually, the low tones disappear as well.

The prevalence of hearing impairment increases after age 50. Hearing loss can be identified in over 33% of persons aged 65 years and older, and in up to half of persons over 85 years. Older persons with hearing impairment are particularly prone to problems such as social and emotional isolation, clinical depression, and limited activity. Many people of all ages suffer from hearing problems. It is also a natural part of the of the aging process.

Auditory Brainstem Response
This test checks the effectiveness of the nervous system in relationship to the ears, and may be utilized in the event of certain types of hearing loss, or if tumors are suspected in the inner ear.

Procedure
The patient's head is hooked up to four electrodes and he is asked to lie down in a darkened room with a set of headphones. A series of tones and clicks is played through the headphones, which often induces sleep in people taking this test. This is normal; the test is measuring the response of the brain to these sounds.

Only 10% of those who could be helped by hearing aids actually wear them. Hearing aid technology has advanced rapidly in recent years, and very small models are available. Telephones and theaters have also designed audio broadcast systems which new hearing aids can pick up.

Results

This test is important because abnormal electrical responses to these simple noises may indicate a tumor in the brain or ear areas. Hearing loss can also be measured with this test.

Electronystagmogram (Caloric Study, ENG)

This test uses different diagnostic tools to study a variety of neurological problems associated with the ears and eyes.

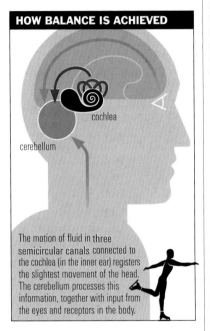

HOW BALANCE IS ACHIEVED

cochlea

cerebellum

The motion of fluid in three semicircular canals connected to the cochlea (in the inner ear) registers the slightest movement of the head. The cerebellum processes this information, together with input from the eyes and receptors in the body.

Procedure

Electrodes are attached to the patient's face, just under each eye and on the bridge of the nose. After the room is darkened, the patient is asked to follow a series of light flashes along a wall. The electrodes record electrical impulses corresponding to eye movement as the lights flash. After that, water, first cold, then warm, is poured into the ears. This stimulates involuntary eye movement (nystagmus). The electrical impulses produced and the movements recorded test the vestibular system of the inner ear, which controls the sense of balance and dizziness. This part of the test may cause nausea and vomiting, because it disturbs the balance centers of the body. There could be problems for patients wearing pacemakers or those with perforated tympanic membranes or those with ventilating tubes in place (for these patients, air is used instead of water).

Nystagmus refers to involuntary rapid movements of the eye in response to certain stimuli. Often these are the result of an abnormality in the balance mechanism of the body, controlled by the inner ear. Usually done on patients who complain of dizziness, this test evaluates the likelihood of a tumor or infection.

Results

Electrical charges caused by eye movement are picked up by electrodes placed near the eyes and recorded on a graph for analysis. Any abnormalities in movement of the eyes or the electrical impulses can be traced to hearing loss, vertigo, or nerve damage, possibly due to brain damage, inflammation or cancer.

5 TOP SUGGESTIONS FOR THOSE WITH HEARING LOSS

1 Consult a doctor.

2 Avoid situations with a lot of background noise.

3 Tell others you have trouble hearing, not to shout, and ask them to repeat or reword what you don't understand.

4 Ask about the availability of amplification earphones at theaters and public events.

5 Always look at the person speaking to you. Even people with normal hearing interpret information from lip movements and facial expressions.

Tympanogram

This test assesses the movement of the tympanic membrane (or eardrum).

more tests ☞

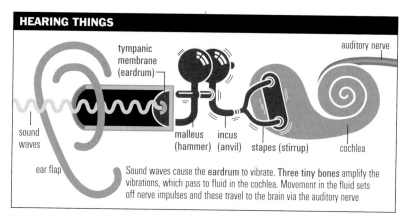

HEARING THINGS

tympanic membrane (eardrum)

auditory nerve

sound waves

ear flap

malleus (hammer)

incus (anvil)

stapes (stirrup)

cochlea

Sound waves cause the **eardrum** to vibrate. **Three tiny bones** amplify the vibrations, which pass to fluid in the cochlea. Movement in the fluid sets off nerve impulses and these travel to the brain via the auditory nerve

Procedure

As in audiometry above, the patient dons headphones. However, these headphones come equipped with a rubber plug, which fits into the ear and up against the eardrum. Pressure is exerted on the plug to test the elasticity of the membrane, which is then recorded by a graphing machine.

Results

Flexibility of the membrane is directly related to its ability to accurately convey sound to the brain. If the graph indicates an abnormal reaction to pressure, it may be the sign of infections, fluid trapped inside the ear, or a perforated eardrum.

NOSE

HOW WE SMELL

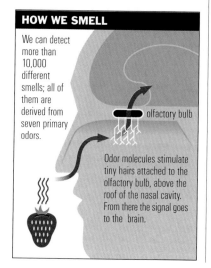

We can detect more than 10,000 different smells; all of them are derived from seven primary odors.

olfactory bulb

Odor molecules stimulate tiny hairs attached to the olfactory bulb, above the roof of the nasal cavity. From there the signal goes to the brain.

Aspiration and Excisional Biopsies

These tests are the beginning of the diagnostic process for serious problems of the sinus.

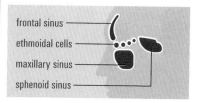

frontal sinus

ethmoidal cells

maxillary sinus

sphenoid sinus

Procedure

These two procedures investigate the sinuses. Both involve a local anesthetic administered to the mouth or nose tissue. In the first, a needle is inserted through the nose and into the sinuses, where it can remove tissue or fluid samples. In the second, tissue samples themselves are cut away from the sinus area. These samples are taken for further examination, such as cultures, blood tests, studies for cancer, etc. There is discomfort involved in having the instruments inserted into the nose and the slight pain of breaking the skin in the sinus area. Bleeding and discomfort may continue for a few days after the tests.

Results

Tests performed on sinus tissue can reveal sinus infections, tumors of the mouth and sinus cavity, as well as many other problems. *See biopsy in the Terms section.*

Allergies result when the immune system overreacts to exposure to a chemical or natural substance. Asthma and hay fever are examples of such allergies. Many allergens are inhaled. Pollen from grass and trees irritates the nose and sinuses, causing runny nose and tearing eyes. Dust and pet shedding can also cause these reactions.

THROAT

Laryngoscopy
This test is a type of endoscopy *(defined in Terms section)* in which the throat is examined for general health or blockage problems.

Procedure
This test is performed under local anesthesia with a laryngoscope, a flexible, tubular instrument about ten inches long. The scope is a complex instrument, and includes fiber optic visualization equipment, a light source and biopsy equipment. Before the test begins, the mouth and throat are anesthetized with a spray. The laryngoscope is inserted either through a nostril or directly into the throat via the mouth. This is slightly uncomfortable, and despite the anesthesia often produces the urge to gag.

Results
The visualization equipment of the scope can show doctors or technicians infections or tumors of the throat and allow a general internal inspection. Other instruments on the scope allow for fluid or tissue collection from the throat area. These samples can be analyzed in a lab for infection and cancerous cells.

Throat Culture
This is a laboratory test of a swab from the throat that is cultured to investigate infection.

THE SWALLOW REFLEX

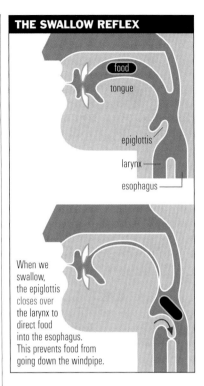

food

tongue

epiglottis

larynx

esophagus

When we swallow, the epiglottis closes over the larynx to direct food into the esophagus. This prevents food from going down the windpipe.

Procedure
A technician inserts a cotton swab deep into the mouth and throat, producing a gag reflex.
This transfers potentially infected mucus and saliva onto the swab, which is then rubbed onto a culture plate. If infection is present, the fluid will grow more bacteria.

Results
This test searches for infection. Growth of certain kinds of bacteria on the culture over a period of time indicates to the doctor that an infection is present, and usually results in the prescription of antibiotics.

Streptococci should be identified in throat cultures, because a specific type of streptococcal pharyngitis (i.e., beta-hemolytic) may be followed by rheumatic heart disease or glomerulonephritis (inflammation of the filtering units of the kidney).

more tests

Excisional Throat Biopsy

This type of biopsy removes a tissue sample from the throat in order to test for infected tissues or tumors.

Procedure

This test may be performed in a doctor's office or in a hospital, but it is always performed under general anesthesia. Once the patient is under anesthesia, the doctor has better access to areas deep in the throat. Using surgical tools, a small tissue sample is removed for biopsy. Once awakened from the anesthesia, the patient may experience soreness and bleeding in the throat for several days. Because of the general anesthesia, the patient should not drive home from the test. This test can take several hours to be performed, and a patient should plan on spending the better part of a day.

Results

The biopsy of the throat seeks infected tissue, or, more likely, tumors or other growths. The biopsy attempts to determine their nature and severity in order to help doctors decide how to proceed. A serious cancer may require surgery and further treatment; a benign cyst may simply be removed.

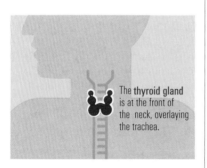

The thyroid gland is at the front of the neck, overlaying the trachea.

Thyroid Stimulating Hormone (TSH) Blood Test

The function of the thyroid is governed by several chemicals in the body, levels of which can be used to predict disease.

Procedure

Blood is drawn from a vein in the arm and subsequently sent to a laboratory to be analyzed.

Results

The presence and quantity of TSH and another hormone, thyroxine, can indicate the beginnings of hypo and hyperthyroidism at levels undetectable in other types of exams.

Radioactive Iodine Uptake (RAI)

This test studies the thyroid's ability to manufacture hormones.

Procedure

After the iodine is administered either orally or intravenously, the patient is asked to lie down on an examination table. Once the iodine has spread through the body, radioactive pictures of the thyroid area are taken over a period of several hours. A gamma camera measures the differences in radiation in various parts of the thyroid, much like a Geiger counter. This test is dangerous to those who are allergic to iodine and shellfish. Since the level of radioactivity is low in the chemicals being used, there is little risk of dangerous exposure.

Results

Iodine is a chemical absorbed almost exclusively by the thyroid, and one which shows up well on these nuclear scans. The pictures measure absorption over time, showing the thyroid's functioning ability. Too much or too little indicates that the thyroid is under- or overactive. This means it may be malfunctioning in its regulation of the metabolism.

Thyroid Radioisotope Scan

This thyroid function test is similar to the one described above.

Procedure

After receiving a radioactive substance (usually orally), the patient lies down on an x-ray table, neck stretched out by a brace. The scanner passes over the patient multiple times and takes pictures of the thyroid area. Unlike the iodine test described above, this not an absorption test over time. Rather, the substance absorbed makes the thyroid stand out clearly in the x-ray pictures. There is no pain involved in this test, and very little radiation risk, as the exposure is very low.

Results

The test is used to evaluate nodules (lumps) in the thyroid. This test may indicate the likelihood of the nodule being benign (harmless) or malignant (cancerous).

TMJ stands for temporomandibular joint, the part of the jaw which connects to the head at the ear. TMJ dysfunction is used to describe chronic pain associated with this joint. This pain can be associated with chewing, grinding of teeth, or other jaw motions. TMJ dysfunction is being diagnosed more and more frequently in the US. Its exact causes and cure are unknown, though many treatments, both invasive and noninvasive, are evolving. Diagnosis is made through a combination of patients' descriptions of symptoms and physical examinations.

For further information

American Academy of Otolaryngology
One Prince Street
Alexandria, VA 22314
(703) 836-4444

American Tinnitus Association
P.O. Box 5
Portland, OR 97207
(800) 634-8978

Thyroid Foundation of America
(800) 832-8321
www.clark.net/pub/tfa

Self Help for Hard of Hearing People, Inc.
7910 Woodmont Avenue
Suite 1200
Bethesda, MD 20814
(301) 657-2248

Every
20 seconds,
a person in the
United States
has a heart
attack.

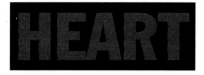

The heart is the muscular pump that beats continuously from before you are born to your last day of life.

It expands and contracts at the rate of 100,000 beats per day, and pumps about 2,000 gallons of blood every twenty-four hours. During an average lifetime, the heart contracts more than 2.5 billion times. Heart tests may be ordered by your primary care physician, or you may be referred to a cardiologist, who specializes in diseases of the heart. **More is known about gender differences involving the heart than any other organ, yet such differentiation is not always recognized in medical diagnostic testing.**

Men's hearts, although larger than women's, beat more slowly, even during sleep.

Advances in the prevention and treatment of heart disease over the past fifty years have been extraordinary, and deaths due to coronary artery disease have decreased 34%.

THE TOP 5 QUESTIONS TO ASK YOUR DOCTOR ABOUT HEART TESTS

? Is this test a routine screening test, or do you see symptoms that cause you to suspect heart disease?

? Is there a less invasive test that can provide you with the same information about my heart?

? What are the possible courses of treatment if the tests indicate evidence of heart disease?

? If the results of my test suggest heart problems, should I be prepared for a hospital stay or surgery?

? What are the risks involved in the particular test being recommended? Radiation? Allergy to dyes? Bleeding? Possible heart attack?

Unfortunately, coronary artery disease is still the number one killer of American men,

and claims the lives of almost twice as men as all forms of cancer put together. Heart disease develops ten years earlier in men than in women—three times more men than women suffer heart attacks before the age of 65. Men also have a 30% greater chance of stroke than women, according to the American Heart Association. Scientists have found that men who smoked fewer than ten cigarettes daily had a 30% higher risk of death from heart disease or lung disease than men who did not smoke. For men who smoke ten cigarettes or more a day, the risk skyrockets to 80%.

New and emerging technologies for treatment of coronary problems, such as external counter-pulsation, transmyocardial laser revascularization, thrombolytic drugs, and the minimally invasive coronary artery bypass surgical techniques (PortCAB, the Octopus system, or the MIDCAB system) are beyond the scope of this book on diagnostics. However, you should consult with your doctor in order to assure that you have the benefit of the latest technology for treatment.

THE TOP 5 WAYS TO REDUCE THE RISK OF HEART DISEASE

 Quit smoking.

 Cut back on foods high in fat, saturated fat and cholesterol.

 Monitor and manage blood pressure and cholesterol levels.

 Exercise regularly at aerobic levels.

 Maintain normal weight for your height.

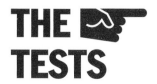

THE TESTS

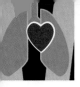

Electrocardiogram (EKG or ECG)

The heart is regulated by electricity. Electrical pulses stimulate the beats of the heart. These pulses, which should be regular in terms of rhythm and frequency, are measured in this test to determine the health of the heart muscle and to identify abnormalities of heart rhythm or rate.

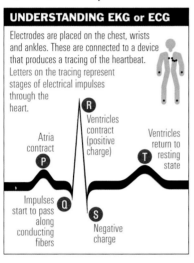

UNDERSTANDING EKG or ECG

Electrodes are placed on the chest, wrists and ankles. These are connected to a device that produces a tracing of the heartbeat. Letters on the tracing represent stages of electrical impulses through the heart.

R — Ventricles contract (positive charge)

Atria contract **P**

Ventricles return to resting state **T**

Impulses start to pass along conducting fibers **Q**

S — Negative charge

Procedure

This test is usually ordered when any symptoms of heart disease—such as chest pain—present themselves, and may be part of a normal physical for patients over certain ages. The patient disrobes from the waist up and lies down. Electrodes are attached to the wrists and ankles with gel. One larger electrode is placed on the chest. This is moved around to different spots near the heart during the test. The test lasts about 15 minutes as the 5 electrodes take amplified readings of the heart's electrical activity. There is no risk of being shocked, and the test is entirely painless.

Results

The results, a 12-line graph, are studied by the doctor. This graph gives a picture of how the heart is working, and can reveal the presence of abnormal rhythms, heart inflammation, and

heart disease. It is an extremely safe, painless diagnostic test, but it gives no indication as to whether a heart attack is imminent. It is, however, useful to compare electrocardiograms done at different times on the same patient, because it can identify warning signs.

Several variations of this test exist. One, called the Holter Monitor, is a 24-hour EKG, which measures the heart throughout an entire day, watching for changes which occur when the body is sleeping, digesting, or moving around, and looking for broader patterns in heart rhythm. Another is called an exercise stress test. During this test, the electrodes are attached as during other EKGs or ECGs, but the patient exercises on a treadmill instead of lying down. This gives readings showing the response of the heart to physical exercise. Additional problems can be detected this way, and this test is often done before a more invasive coronary angiograph with cardiac catheterization is performed.

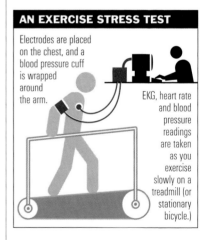

AN EXERCISE STRESS TEST

Electrodes are placed on the chest, and a blood pressure cuff is wrapped around the arm.

EKG, heart rate and blood pressure readings are taken as you exercise slowly on a treadmill (or stationary bicycle.)

Chest X-Ray

This plain x-ray can identify many problems in general, although specific information about the heart is often sought. It searches for abnormal heart size or lung congestion (heart failure),

ANATOMY OF A HEARTBEAT

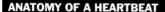

In a cycle that repeats about 70 times a minute, heart muscles pump blood through the heart into the body.

1 Diastole

Atria and ventricles dilate; blood flows into them.

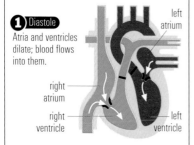

left atrium

right atrium

right ventricle

left ventricle

2 Atrial systole

The atria contract, pushing any remaining blood into the ventricles.

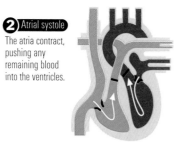

3 Ventricular systole

The ventricles contract, sending blood from the heart to the lungs and the rest of the body.

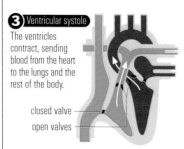

closed valve

open valves

lung problems (pneumonia, blood clot, tumors) and rib cage abnormalities (cancer, broken bones) in the upper chest.

Procedure

The patient undresses from the waist up and stands next to the x-ray plate. A lead screen may be provided to cover the genitalia to protect them from exposure to radiation. The x-ray camera is aimed at the chest and the pictures taken. The film is then removed from the x-ray plate to be developed, which takes only a short while. To evaluate the heart, a frontal and side view are usually obtained.

Results

The heart, lungs and ribs are all visible in this type of x-ray. Broken or otherwise abnormal ribs can be seen, as can large tumors, clots or fluid in the lungs. Emphysema can also be diagnosed based on the results. Abnormal heart size or shape may be seen as well.

Echocardiogram

This ultrasound test can give an accurate picture of the structure and inner workings of the heart in motion with considerable accuracy and without the radiation of an x-ray.

Procedure

The patient lies down on a table, removes clothing from the waist up, and a gel is spread on the chest which will help transmit sound waves. The transducer, the pen-like instrument used in all ultrasounds, is passed over the heart area of the chest until a good spot can be found. The technician moves the transducer around the heart area for approximately half an hour, taking readings.

Results

The sound waves bouncing from the transducer to the body and back can be converted into both pictures and graphs. The pictures are like a video of the inside of the heart as it beats. The doctor can determined the internal size of the heart chamber, the thickness of the chamber walls, whether there is excess fluid building up around the heart, contractile power of the heart muscle, and whether the four valves of the heart are narrowed, inflamed or leaking. The main value of an echocardiogram is in identifying abnormalities of heart valves, and in calculating a number called the "ejection fraction," which is useful in diagnosing heart failure. The "ejection fraction" is the percent of blood in the heart that is pumped out with a single beat.

more tests

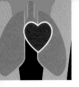

Coronary Angiography with Cardiac Catheterization

An angiogram is a specialized x-ray which is done by injecting radiopaque dye (a radioactive substance) into the blood vessels leading to the heart in order to visualize abnormalities (narrowing of the arteries). Structural abnormalities in the heart absorb the dye at different rates, and thus the x-rays identify these structures. While angiography is used in blood vessels outside the heart, it is particularly useful with the heart and the blood vessels through which it pumps blood.

Cardiac catheterization is one of the greatest advances in cardiology in recent medical history. It is a test that is performed when coronary artery disease is suspected, and is used to decide whether or not surgery is necessary.

BLOCKED BLOOD SUPPLY

When a coronary artery is partially or completely blocked...

...heart muscle dies, because it has an inadequate blood supply.

Procedure

The test is done in a special room, usually in a hospital, and requires a fair amount of preparation by the patient, including fasting from the previous night and taking a sedative. Electrocardiogram (EKG or ECG) monitors will be attached to the patient to measure heart rate and rhythm while the test is going on. A thin catheter is inserted into a vein or artery of the body, usually in the upper leg/groin area, after this area

has been anesthetized with an injection. The catheter is guided through the body into the heart itself. The catheter can also be used to take pressure readings, collect blood, and inject dye into the heart. (Less commonly, dye is simply injected into a blood vessel.) As the dye spreads through the body to the area of interest (specific blood vessels or the heart) x-rays are taken of that area. Although an important diagnostic tool, this procedure does involve risk. Approximately 1 in 1000 patients die of a heart attack during or after the procedure. However, the risk of dying from a cardiac event for high risk patients is much greater than the risk of death during the procedure.

Results

This test is usually performed following an EKG or ECG, Echocardiogram and stress test. The doctor can clearly see clogged arteries or malfunctioning heart tissue with this test, both at the end of the catheter and through the x-rays that can be obtained. This can lead the doctor to decide about bypass surgery, angioplasty, revascularization procedures or drug therapy.

Nuclear Heart Scans: Thallium, Stress-Thallium, Technetium

The nuclear scan is important in diagnosing heart disease. This test can measure the health of heart tissues, as well as provide images of heart function.

Procedure

One of several nuclear isotopes is injected into the body. All isotopes are absorbed differently as the blood moves through the heart, depending on damage to it. Shortly after injection, the gamma camera is used to photograph the heart.

Results

The pictures from this test can detect whether areas of heart tissue have

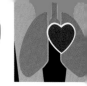

died during a heart attack. The doctor can also see if some areas of the heart are not getting sufficient oxygen or are not pumping properly. This often causes the painful condition known as angina. The doctor may order additional tests, such as angiography with cardiac catheterization after seeing these results. This test replaces the exercise stress test in patients for whom exercise poses great risk.

Electron Beam Computed Tomography (EBCT) or Ultrafast CT

This relatively new noninvasive test is able to accurately determine the amount of calcium content in coronary arteries, which some medical experts believe may be a predictor of heart disease.

Procedure

Utilizing a specialized type of Ultrafast CT scanner with electron beams, the patient is asked to lie on a large tray which slides into the scanner. The scan may require twenty to thirty minutes, during which the patient is requested to lie still. The procedure is entirely painless, but will expose the patient to higher levels of radiation than a normal x-ray series, although well within medically acceptable limits.

Results

Because this electron beam technique allows the technicians to take higher speed images, they can capture x-ray pictures of the moving vessels as the heart is beating. EBCT scanning is promising as a preventive tool because the test is painless, noninvasive, and risk free. However, it is considered a controversial emerging technology with a high rate of false positive and negative results. Also, experts disagree about whether or not calcium deposits in the arteries are accurate predictors of future risk of coronary artery disease.

SIGNS OF HEART DISEASE

- Chest discomfort,
- Shortness of breath,
- Fatigue and
- Palpitations and
- Dizziness.

RISK FACTORS INCLUDE

- Hypertension
- Diabetes
- Elevated cholesterol
- Smoking
- Obesity
- Lack of physical activity.

Blood tests for lipids/cholesterol, triglycerides, HDL, LDL

Lipid is a term for any fat in the bloodstream. Excess buildup of lipids can clog arteries and cause heart attacks and strokes. Blood tests for lipids evaluate risk of heart disease, clogged arteries, diabetes and pancreatitis (in the case of triglycerides). Taken over time, they also measure the effect of exercise on fat in the blood.

Procedure

Blood is drawn after the patient has been fasting, and is sent to a lab for analysis.

Results

Many measurements return from a lipid test. Cholesterol is a fatty compound which is produced in the body and is necessary in small quantities, but can build up and clog arteries when blood levels are high. Triglycerides are the most dominant lipid in the body, and have some correlation to heart disease. Low Density Lipoprotein (LDL) is often referred to as the "bad" or dangerous cholesterol product. High Density

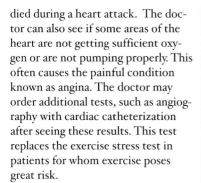

more tests ☞

Lipoprotein (HDL) is the beneficial or "good" cholesterol, and has an inverse relationship to heart disease: high HDL decreases the risk. LDL is the opposite: high LDL increases the risk of heart disease.

Apolipoproteins Blood Test

Apolipoproteins—the protein fractions of lipoprotein molecules—are an important component of the blood. They may indicate the patient's risk of coronary artery disease.

Procedure

Blood is taken from a vein and sent to a lab for analysis.

Results

High levels of the lipoprotein are indicative of potential risk of coronary artery disease, among other illnesses.

Blood Test for Heart Enzyme, CPK (creatine phosphokinase), CK (creatine kinase), SGOT (serum glutamic-oxaloacetic transaminase), LDH (lactate dehydrogenase)

These are all substances which exist in muscle, including heart muscle, and leak into the blood when a heart attack or other damage has occurred. Elevated levels in the bloodstream can indicate such damage. This test often accompanies an EKG test in order to diagnose heart attacks.

Procedure

Blood is drawn from a vein and sent to a lab for analysis. Sometimes this test is done immediately after a patient is admitted with chest pain, so the circumstances may vary.

Results

If elevated levels of CPK, LDH or CK are found in the bloodstream, they may have come from damaged heart, brain or muscle cells. More specific tests can

be done to localize these enzymes, which leak for up to two days after a heart attack.

SGOT is found in both the liver and the heart, and is always found in measurable amounts in the bloodstream.

No one of these enzymes is definitive evidence of heart damage, but they are examined in conjunction with an EKG to assist in diagnosis. These tests are sometimes repeated over several hours to determine if an evolving pattern of muscle damage can be identified.

Blood Test for Vitamin B1

A poor diet can result in vitamin deficiencies. Although this test is not specific to or diagnostic of heart disease, a lack of vitamin B1 can be particularly dangerous to the heart.

Procedure

Blood is drawn from a vein and sent to a lab for analysis. Fasting is required before the tests so that vitamin-rich foods do not adversely affect the outcome.

Results

A low level of the vitamin, usually due to poor diet, can lead to muscle weakness and potentially to heart failure. If found, vitamin deficiency is usually treated with vitamin supplements.

Hematocrit Blood Test

This general blood test measures red blood cells as a percentage of total blood volume in a sample (see Complete Blood Count), but this test is not specific to or diagnostic of heart disease.

Procedure

Blood is drawn from a vein or from a finger prick for analysis. The hematocrit is simply the measure of the height of the column of red blood

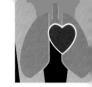

cells after a blood sample goes through a centrifuge, which separates blood into its parts.

Results

A low reading can indicate anemia, while an abnormally high reading can mean poor oxygenation of the blood, which occurs commonly in certain kinds of congenital heart disease and in emphysema.

Blood Test for Antimyocardial Antibodies

Some chemicals within the body are confined within an organ unless the organ is damaged. At that point, these compounds leak into the bloodstream or urine.

Procedure

Blood is drawn from a vein and taken to a lab for analysis.

Results

These antibodies may be present in the blood in cases of rheumatic heart disease or certain kinds of weakness of the heart muscle.

For Further Information:

American Heart Association
7272 Greenville Avenue
Dallas, TX 75231
214-373-6300
www.americanheart.org

Center for Cardiovascular Education
www.heartinfo.org

LUNGS

The lungs are the main organ of the respiratory system. They supply the body with oxygen (O_2) and eliminate carbon dioxide (CO_2). Some tests on the lungs may be ordered by your personal physician. You may be referred to a pulmonologist, a doctor with several years of specialized training in diseases of the lungs. These diseases may be acute (many resulting from an immediate condition such as pneumonia) or chronic, having to do with exposure to a given problem over time (such as emphysema from cigarette smoke).

Lung disease is the number three cause of death in the United States, responsible for one in every seven deaths.

THE TOP 6 QUESTIONS TO ASK YOUR DOCTOR ABOUT LUNG TESTS

? If I have a problem breathing, what should I do right away?

? What is the best test to diagnose my particular symptoms?

? Are there any conditions that would make a test a bad idea?

? Are there any restrictions on my diet or activities before the test?

? Does the clinic or hospital require a patient consent form in order to take this test?

? How will I feel after the test?

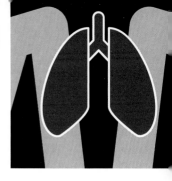

Lung cancer affects many more men than women—there were 772,000 new cases among men in 1998, compared with 265,000 new cases among women. Cigarette smoking is the main cause of lung cancer. A total of 93% of all lung cancer deaths in 1995 were attributed to smoking. **Men who smoke are approximately ten times more likely to develop lung cancer than nonsmoking men.**

Tobacco use is also a major risk factor for other cancers, such as esophageal (food pipe) and throat cancer, as well as other respiratory problems such as emphysema and chronic bronchitis. A man who smokes is two to six times more likely to suffer a heart attack than a nonsmoking man, and the risk increases with the number of cigarettes smoked each day. Unfortunately, approximately 47 million Americans are smokers.

Asthma, an important lung condition, affects approximately 5% of the population. Between the ages of 20 to 50, men account for one third of asthma-related hospital admissions.

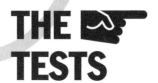

THE TESTS

Arterial blood gases

This blood test is not performed routinely. For patients with potentially more serious lung conditions, it measures levels of oxygen, carbon dioxide, and acid in the blood in order to determine lung function. Abnormal levels of the various gases may indicate the lungs are failing to bring oxygen in and expel CO_2 properly, suggesting lung disease.

Procedure

Because this test is slightly more difficult than other blood tests, blood must be obtained from an artery rather than from a vein. Arteries are usually found deeper in the arm than veins. The blood sample is then sent to a lab for analysis. This test is often performed on patients whose lung function is in question, or before surgery.

Results

Lung disease and heart disease often go hand-in-hand. The lung's function is to remove CO_2 and put oxygen into the blood. The heart's job is to pump the blood to the entire body, where oxygen is delivered to tissues and CO_2 is picked up for expulsion. Blood gases by themselves are not indicators of specific diseases. However, abnormal blood gas levels are an important indicator of how well the heart and lungs are functioning, and can provide important information in making a diagnosis.

Carboxyhemoglobin

Acute carbon monoxide exposure is often deadly. In addition, long-term exposure at low levels, which can occur at factories or in some homes, can cause serious medical problems. The carboxyhemoglobin test is a measure of carbon monoxide in the blood, which can be used to explain symptoms.

Procedure

Blood is drawn from a vein and sent to a lab for analysis. This test is not done very often, but may be ordered for those who complain of fatigue and headache which are suspected to be environment-related.

Results

The result is expressed in a percentage of carboxyhemoglobin in the blood. Carbon monoxide attaches or bonds to hemoglobin (the oxygen-carrying pigment found in red blood cells), preventing it from carrying oxygen, which is why it is so dangerous. If more than 5% of hemoglobin is found to have carbon monoxide, it is likely that some external factor is contributing the gas to the body.

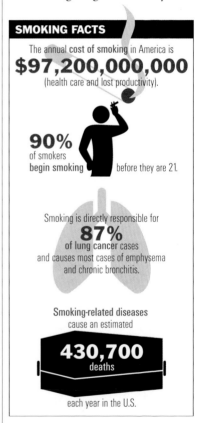

SMOKING FACTS

The annual cost of smoking in America is

$97,200,000,000

(health care and lost productivity).

90%
of smokers
begin smoking   before they are 21.

Smoking is directly responsible for
87%
of lung cancer cases
and causes most cases of emphysema
and chronic bronchitis.

Smoking-related diseases
cause an estimated

430,700
deaths

each year in the U.S.

Pulmonary Function Test (PFT or Spirometry)

Lungs constantly inflate and deflate as we breathe. There are many measures of the "mechanics" of breathing.

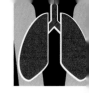

When abnormal, these can point to certain diagnoses. Examples of these measures include how much air is taken in with one breath, how fast it can be expelled and how much is left after letting the breath out.

Procedure

This test simply involves breathing down a tube into a machine which measures lung capacity and strength. The patient is given a mouthpiece attached to a machine and is instructed to breathe into it normally, inhale or exhale deeply, or perform similar tasks.

Results

The results of this test are measured on an instrument called a spirogram. Results can be used to diagnose diseases such as asthma and emphysema, or to see how these diseases are affecting breathing ability.

Bronchogram

Although this x-ray is not needed frequently, it is designed to get a clearer picture of the lungs than a normal chest x-ray can provide.

Procedure

This test requires a considerable amount of patient preparation, including fasting and taking both a sedative as well as a medication to decrease mucus production. The mouth is also anesthetized or "numbed" with a spray or swab, and anesthetic drops are placed deeper into the throat. A plastic tube called a catheter is inserted through the mouth into the lungs. Contrast material (which shows up on an x-ray) is injected into the lungs through the catheter, where the progress of breathing distributes it throughout the lungs. X-rays are then taken of the lungs. This test often induces a lot of coughing.

Results

The contrast material outlines the airway tubes, and shows up on an x-ray. The appearance of the x-rays can help make a diagnosis.

Bronchoscopy

This is a type of endoscopy that uses a special camera that can go around narrow passages in order to actually look directly at the tissues inside the bronchial tubes. It can also be used to remove an object lodged in the windpipe or to take a biopsy.

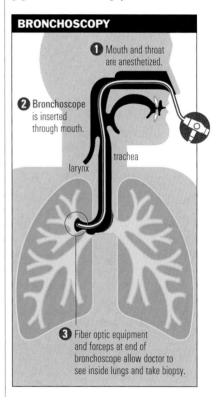

BRONCHOSCOPY

1 Mouth and throat are anesthetized.

2 Bronchoscope is inserted through mouth.

trachea

larynx

3 Fiber optic equipment and forceps at end of bronchoscope allow doctor to see inside lungs and take biopsy.

Procedure

As with the bronchogram, the mouth and throat are anesthetized. The patient takes a sedative and is given other medication to decrease secretions. The bronchoscope, a flexible tube, is inserted through the mouth, down the windpipe and into the bronchial tubes. At the end is fiber optic visualization equipment and biopsy equipment. A biopsy can be obtained with forceps that actually cut a piece of tissue, or with a brush that gathers cells for collection. This

more tests ◢

test sometimes involves a certain degree of discomfort and anxiety. (That is why a sedative is given.) The patient should arrange to be driven home after this test. The test provides a pulmonologist with the most direct information possible about the condition of the tissues.

Results

Sometimes an x-ray of the bronchial tubes and lungs cannot not reveal small problems. This test allows the doctor to look directly into the area and observe closely any tumors, clots or foreign objects lodged in these areas. Biopsies can be performed on the tissue and blood and fluid samples can also be taken. This procedure is primarily used to diagnose tumors.

ASTHMA

An estimated 14.6 million persons in the United States have asthma, a condition marked by coughing and difficulty in breathing. An asthma attack, which can be triggered by smoke, pet hair, pollen or other allergies, respiratory infections, exercise or strong odors, is a narrowing or thickening of the bronchial tubes which lead to the lungs. Its cause is not understood, but several types of treatment can control most asthma attacks effectively. Still, 5,600 American people die of asthma every year. Approximately 33% of asthma patients are under the age of 18. It is the most common chronic illness among children.

Mediastinoscopy

This endoscopy is performed less often than bronchoscopy. It is performed through an incision in the chest. Rather than examining the lungs directly, a scope called a mediastinoscope is used to directly examine the lymph nodes and other tissue which surround the lungs.

Procedure

A mediastinoscopy is performed under general anesthesia. The patient is put to sleep in an operating room, and an incision is made in the notch at the top of the ribcage. The endoscope is inserted and can withdraw fluid, allow visualizations, or obtain tissue samples, including lymph nodes. This test involves some risk, as does any procedure under general anesthesia.

Results

While this test draws fluid and can take pictures just as other endoscopies, it is usually ordered to get a biopsy of lymph node tissue. Doctors may suspect cancer of the lymph nodes or lungs, which can be detected with a biopsy. Some other diseases of the lung, such as tuberculosis, can also be diagnosed through this procedure.

Sputum culture

Sputum is the name given to any material that is expelled from the lungs. Thus, it is more than just saliva and mucus. This material is tested for evidence of infection by being cultured for bacteria, tuberculosis or other organisms.

Procedure

The patient coughs up sputum into a cup, which is taken to a lab for analysis. A mist which promotes coughing may be administered to stimulate production of sputum.

Results

An analysis of sputum can help diagnose pneumonia and bronchitis and, most importantly, tuberculosis.

Influenza and pneumonia combined are the sixth leading cause of death in the United States.

Thoracentesis

The lungs sit in what is called the "chest cavity." Sometimes abnormal amounts of fluid can collect in the

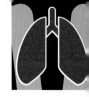

small space between the lungs and the chest cavity wall. A thoracentesis withdraws this fluid from the chest for analysis.

THORACENTESIS

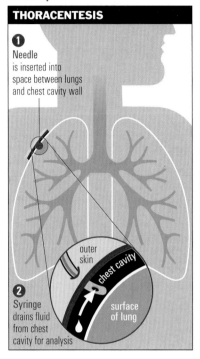

❶
Needle
is inserted into
space between lungs
and chest cavity wall

outer skin

chest cavity

❷
Syringe
drains fluid
from chest
cavity for analysis

surface
of lung

Procedure
A small area of the chest is injected with a local anesthetic. Then, a needle is inserted and is positioned into the space where the fluid has collected. Fluid is removed with a syringe for analysis. If needed, a larger amount can be drained if it is causing discomfort or intruding on normal body functions such as breathing. This test can be performed in the doctor's office and should last not more than approximately 30 minutes. The patient should arrange to be driven home after this test.

Results
The analysis from the lab reports on the content of the fluid. This can include protein, glucose, bacteria, and cancerous cells. Fluid around the lungs can indicate lung cancer and pneumonia, as well as other chest abnormalities or infections.

Lung scan
There are two types of this nuclear scan, which tests for blood clots in the lung, abnormal oxygen absorption and lung function.

Procedure
In the first type of test, a radioactive substance is injected into a vein and spreads to the lungs. A "gamma camera" then takes pictures of the lungs. In the second type, the patient inhales a gas containing radioisotopes into the lungs and pictures are then taken. The radioisotope is not dangerous in the small amount given.

Results
The radioactive substance injected into the vein will not spread to areas of the lung where blood vessels are blocked by blood clots. Thus, areas with clots will not show up on the nuclear scan pictures. The pictures from the gas test demonstrate which parts of the lung are effectively exchanging air. If the gas does not absorb into some parts of the lung, it means those parts are not working properly. Both types of lung scan, together called a "ventilation-perfusion" lung scan, are most commonly performed in patients in whom a blood clot is suspected.

For Further Information

The American Lung Association
432 Park Avenue South
8th Floor
New York, NY 10016
1-800-LUNG-USA (1-800-586-4872)
www.lungusa.org

Asthma In America Survey Project
1901 L Street NW
Suite 300
Washington, DC 20036
(202) 452-9429
(202) 296-3727 fax
www.asthmainamerica.com

The liver processes about six cups of blood each minute, extracting nutrients and oxygen.

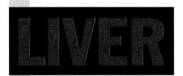

LIVER

The liver is the largest solid organ in the body.

It weighs between 2.5 and 3.3 pounds and is about the size of a football. It manufactures the majority of chemicals in the body, and regulates the levels of most of the main chemicals in the blood. It converts glucose into material that can be stored and used later. It also breaks down fats and proteins, and produces enzymes necessary for blood clotting. It processes bile, a necessary ingredient to digestion, and filters drugs and alcohol out of the body. Although the liver is quite complex in its functions, it is not delicate. **The liver is so durable that up to 75% of its cells can be destroyed or surgically removed before it ceases to function.** Though it is not fragile, its complexities make it extremely important to the overall function of the body.

Disorders of the liver include hepatitis (liver inflammation), cancer, tumors, cysts, bile duct/gallbladder diseases and cirrhosis. **Cirrhosis** is a name for any of a multitude of chronic diseases which stress the liver and over time cause scarring. Cirrhosis is simply scarring that results from liver damage. Cirrhosis prevents proper blood flow to the liver, so that it cannot continue to produce the proteins and other necessary substances the body needs. It also slows the ability of the liver to process nutrients and toxins. Most commonly associated with alcoholism, cirrhosis is the seventh leading cause of death by disease overall. For Americans between

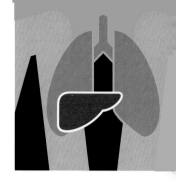

the ages of 25 and 44, it is the fourth largest disease-related cause of death. **Liver disease due to excessive consumption of alcohol outnumbers all other types of liver disorder by five to one.** CT scans can be used to detect cirrhosis and other liver disorders. The liver can also be biopsied.

Hepatitis may be caused by viral infection, alcohol abuse, chemicals, or prescription drugs. Various strains of viral hepatitis from A through G and GB have been identified. All can be damaging to the liver. Hepatitis A and B are preventable with vaccines and controllable. **There are an estimated 3.9 million Americans with Hepatitis C, for which there is no vaccine and no definitive treatment.** (A cocktail of Interferon and Ribavirin has shown promising results in treating Hepatitis C, but this treatment is still being tested.) Liver damage due to Hepatitis C is the leading cause of liver transplants in the United States.

For hepatitis, preventive measures and early detection through testing are the best protection.

THE TOP 5 WAYS TO BE GOOD TO YOUR LIVER

- Don't drink excessive amounts of alcohol.
- Avoid foods high in fats.
- Drink 6 to 8 glasses of water daily.
- Maintain normal weight for your height.
- Maintain abdominal muscle tone.

THE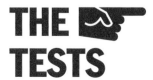
TESTS

IT'S ABOUT THE SIZE OF A FOOTBALL

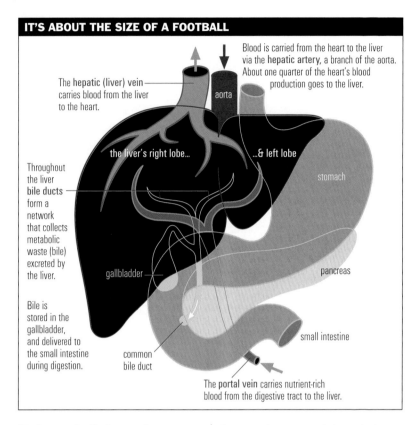

The **hepatic (liver) vein** carries blood from the liver to the heart.

Blood is carried from the heart to the liver via the **hepatic artery**, a branch of the aorta. About one quarter of the heart's blood production goes to the liver.

aorta

the liver's right lobe...

...& left lobe

stomach

Throughout the liver **bile ducts** form a network that collects metabolic waste (bile) excreted by the liver.

gallbladder

pancreas

Bile is stored in the gallbladder, and delivered to the small intestine during digestion.

common bile duct

small intestine

The **portal vein** carries nutrient-rich blood from the digestive tract to the liver.

Endoscopic Retrograde Cholangiopancreatography (ERCP)

The bile ducts connect the liver to the small intestine through a small opening called the ampulla of Vater in order to distribute bile for digestion. An endoscope, inserted via the mouth, examines the liver via this opening, and is particularly useful for taking successful x-rays of the bile ducts in order to determine the presence of cancer, infection, blockage with gallstones, scarring, or some obstruction within the bile duct. Cancer of the pancreas may also be diagnosed with this procedure.

Procedure

The patient fasts for 12 hours before the test, so that the intestine will be as clear as possible. The mouth and throat may be anesthetized, and a sedative is often given as well. The endoscope, about the diameter of a finger, is then inserted through the mouth and guided into the stomach and small intestine. The endoscope can enter the ampulla and usually does so to inject dye into the bile ducts. X-rays are then taken of the liver area, and other endoscopic procedures can be performed. These include removal of stones from the bile duct area. Because of the use of anesthesia and possibly sedatives, the patient should be driven home after this test.

Results

The x-rays of the liver area should be very clear because of the dye injected. Bile duct infections and blockages should be visible. Because the scope allows detailed inspection of this area of the body, other problems or blockages may be revealed. The material removed from the biopsy can be tested for cancers or infections. This test is safer than exploratory surgery and may provide the same result.

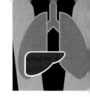

Abdominal Ultrasound

This ultrasound can be used to evaluate the liver, aorta, kidney, gallbladder, lymph nodes, uterus and ovaries, and other solid organs in the abdomen. The intestines, however, do not show up well on the ultrasound.

Procedure

The patient disrobes from the waist up and lies down on an examination table. A gel is put on the abdomen to help transmit sound waves. The technician then moves the transducer over the parts of the abdomen which are of importance to the doctor.

Results

Like other ultrasound results, these appear on a screen which can be studied by the doctor. This test reads gallstones and kidney stones especially well. It can detect inflammations and also differentiate between solid and fluid-filled masses, useful for examining suspected tumors. It is helpful in identifying masses outside the liver or gallbladder compressing these organs. Depending on the results of the ultrasound, the doctor may request a biopsy of the organs involved.

Each year, more than 25 million Americans suffer from liver and gallbladder diseases, and more than 43,000 die of liver disease annually.

Computed Tomography of the Biliary Tract and Liver (Liver CT Scan)

Multiple x-ray scans of the biliary tract and liver are reconstructed by computer as two-dimensional images on a monitor. Sometimes a contrast medium is used to accentuate differences in tissue density.

Procedure

The patient is asked to lie down on an x-ray table, and the table is positioned in the opening of a scanning gantry. If a contrast medium is taken orally, the patient may be asked to fast until after the test. If a contrast medium is introduced intravenously, no fasting is necessary. The scanning process can take as long as an hour, during which the patient is requested to remain as motionless as possible.

Ultrasonography is often performed on the liver instead of CT because it is less expensive and does not expose the patient to radiation. The CT scan usually provides a level of detail that ultrasound cannot.

Results

The size, shape and function of the liver can be observed from the CT. Cysts, tumors and abscesses will show up on the CT.

Percutaneous Liver Biopsy

Under local anesthesia, a special hypodermic needle is inserted through the chest wall into the liver, and a sample of tissue is drawn out by aspiration. This sample allows medical specialists to determine the health of the liver tissue.

Procedure

The patient is asked to lie down and to remain as still as possible. An anesthetic is injected, and when the area is sufficiently anesthetized, the patient is asked to take a deep breath, exhale, and hold his breath at the end of the expiration. A special needle with a flange to control depth of penetration, called a Menghini needle is used to penetrate the upper abdominal wall and the liver, and, using the plunger of the syringe, to aspirate a small specimen of tissue into the tip of the needle. This process should take place in a few seconds, but the patient is usually required to remain resting under the doctor's observation for two hours. Under certain circumstances, the needle may require guidance to a particular place in the

more tests

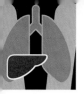

liver, in which case, CT scanning or ultrasound may be performed simultaneously with the biopsy.

Results

The specimen of tissue must be transported to the laboratory for analysis immediately. Examination of the tissue will reveal signs of cirrhosis, hepatitis, or infections such as tuberculosis. Tissue analysis will also identify various forms of cancer, as well as non-cancerous tumors.

Mono Spot Blood Test

This blood test for mononucleosis, a debilitating illness that swells the liver and spleen, enables the doctor to make a definitive diagnosis. Mono, which often occurs in teenagers and young adults, manifests itself in extreme fatigue, prolonged headache, strong fever and sore throat.

Procedure

Blood is drawn from a vein and sent to a lab for analysis.

Results

If the test comes back positive, another confirming test may be performed.

Alanine Aminotransferase Blood Test (ALT) or Serum Glutamic-Pyruvic Transminase Blood Test (SGPT)

Injury or disease in the liver causes leakage of this enzyme into the bloodstream. The most likely diseases causing this leakage are hepatitis, mononucleosis or acute injury with infection, drugs or alcohol.

Procedure

Blood is drawn from a vein and sent to a lab for analysis.

Results

An elevated level of ALT in the blood is a sign of liver inflammation.

WHY ALCOHOL ABUSE IS BAD FOR YOUR LIVER

1 Most alcohol is converted by enzymes in the liver into **acetaldehyde** which, like alcohol itself, is toxic to liver cells.

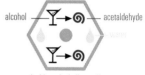

alcohol — acetaldehyde

inside a single liver cell

2 Acetaldehyde causes **alcoholic hepatitis**, which inflames and damages liver cells and the liver's ability to function.

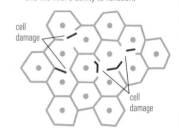

cell damage

cell damage

3 Alcohol abuse also causes fat to accumulate in liver cells, a condition called **fatty liver**.

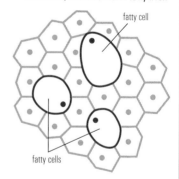

fatty cell

fatty cells

4 If people with alcoholic hepatitis or fatty liver continue to abuse alcohol, **cirrhosis**, which is irreversible, can develop.

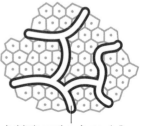

In cirrhosis, **scar tissue** forms on the liver, separating cells into clumps.

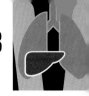

More than 25,000 Americans die each year from cirrhosis of the liver, the seventh leading cause of death.

Alpha-fetoprotein Blood Test (AFP)

AFP is a protein produced by the fetal liver and yolk sac. Increased levels of AFP may indicate liver tumors.

Procedure

Blood is drawn from a vein and sent to a lab for analysis.

Results

This compound is elevated in the blood of patients with liver and other cancers, in particular, testicular cancer. It can also be elevated by cirrhosis or chronic active hepatitis.

Alkaline Phosphatase Blood Test (ALP)

Although ALP is found in many tissues, it is particularly concentrated in the liver and the biliary tract epithelium. Detection of this enzyme is important for determining liver and bone disorders.

Procedure

Blood is taken from a vein and sent to a lab for analysis.

Results

Elevated levels of this compound in the bloodstream may indicate cirrhosis, obstruction of the bile duct, or a liver tumor.

Bilirubin Blood Test

Bilirubin results from the breakdown of blood cells by the liver, which then eliminates them from the body via the intestines. Too much bilirubin in the body means that blood cells are not being eliminated properly. This can cause jaundice, a yellowing of the skin.

Procedure

Blood is taken from a vein and sent to a lab for analysis. This test is often done in conjunction with a number of other tests, known as liver function tests.

Results

Excessive red blood cell destruction from disease leads to elevated bilirubin. Blockage of the bile ducts from cancer, gallstones, or scarring can also cause elevated bilirubin.

TYPES OF HEPATITIS

A preventable by vaccine; unpleasant but has no lasting effects

B preventable by vaccine; potentially fatal if untreated; controllable with drugs

C no vaccine; extremely dangerous; no definitive cure or control

D rare; only exists as coinfection with Hepatitis B; accelerates liver damage

E extremely rare in U.S.; no chronic liver disease

F extremely rare in U.S.; not sufficiently studied

G blood borne viral infection; long-term effects unknown

Hepatitis B and C can be transmitted by receiving blood transfusions, but today that is rare. The most common causes now are contaminated drug injections and unprotected sex. The most obvious sign of the disease is jaundice, a yellowing of the skin.

Protein, Albumin, Serum Protein, Globulin and Serum Electrophoresis Blood Tests

These proteins are essential to the liver's function as the body's "factory."

Procedure

Blood is drawn from a vein and sent to a lab for analysis.

more tests ▶

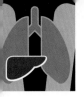

Results
Serum protein is high in patients with cirrhosis and leukemia. Low albumin is a sign of kidney disease, edema or fluid in the lungs. Decreased levels of the other proteins are signs of malnutrition, starvation, liver disease, or cancer.

Hepatitis Blood Test
Viral hepatitis, caused by a damaging virus, is the second most common problem with the liver, behind alcoholic liver disease. Hepatitis A is transmitted by eating uncooked food or drinking unsanitary water. It is quite contagious, inflames the liver, and also causes fatigue and muscle aches, but does no permanent damage to the liver. Hepatitis B and C, however, are spread through contact with contaminated blood and are much more dangerous, often leading to cirrhosis or other liver failure. Both B and C also can be transmitted sexually (see also Reproductive Organs).

Procedure
Blood is drawn from a vein and sent to a lab for analysis.

Results
Blood can be tested for the presence of the virus or antibodies to it. Since there is a vaccine for A and B, these antibodies can result in a false positive test. Hepatitis can only be controlled, not cured, with drugs.

Ammonia Level Blood and Urine Test
Ammonia is generated by bacteria acting on proteins present in the digestive system. It then moves to the liver, where it is normally converted into urea and then secreted through the kidneys.

Procedure
A blood sample is taken from a vein and sent to a lab for analysis. If a urine test is required as well, a urine sample is gathered.

Results
Ammonia is always present in blood and urine, but in high quantities indicate severe liver disease.

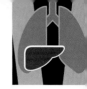

For Further Information

American Liver Foundation
75 Maiden Lane, Suite #603
New York, NY 10038
1-800-GO LIVER (1-800-465-4837)
www.gi.ucsf.edu/ALF/

National Network for Organ Sharing
1100 Boulders Parkway, Suite #500
P.O. Box 13770
Richmond, VA 23225-8770
1-804-330-8500

American Association for the Study
of Liver Diseases
www.hepar-sfgh.ucsf.edu

Johns Hopkins Division of Infectious
Diseases: Hepatitis
www.hopkins-id.edu/diseases/
hepatitis

American Gastrointestinal
Association
www.gastro.org

National Center for Infectious
Diseases (CDC): Viral Hepatitis
1-888-4-HEP-CDC (1-888-443-7232)
www.cdc.gov/ncidod/diseases/
hepatitis/index.htm

The kidneys filter approximately 40 gallons of blood daily.

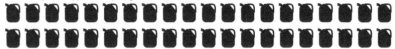

Each kidney
is about
4 inches long
(the size shown here)
and weighs
6 ounces.

KIDNEYS

The kidneys, ureter, bladder, and urethra comprise the urinary tract. Kidneys remove liquid waste from the blood in the form of urine, keep a stable balance of salts and other substances in the blood, regulate blood pressure, and produce erythroprotein, a hormone that aids in the formation of red blood cells. **A nephrologist is a specialist who deals with diseases of the kidneys.** Depending on the nature of the complaint or test ordered, a patient may also be referred to **a urologist, who treats problems with the urinary tract once urine has left the kidneys.**

Within the kidney, microscopic units called nephrons filter waste products from the blood.

The efficiency of the kidney diminishes with age as the number of functional nephrons declines. Kidney disorders include kidney cancer, congenital disorders, glomerulonephritis (an inflammation of the nephrons), and kidney stones. Diabetes and high blood pressure are also common causes of kidney damage. **Kidney stones** are one of the most common disorders of the urinary tract, and are extremely painful. Blood in the urine is a frequent sign. Kidney stones occur more frequently in men than in women. They develop from crystals, usually made largely of calcium, which form in the urine. Approximately 10% of all Americans will develop a kidney stone, although most pass out of the body without a doctor's intervention. **Kidney stones strike people most often between the ages of 20 and 40.** However, once a person gets more than one stone, he is more likely to develop others. Kidney stones are usually detected through urinalysis, which can be confirmed with an x-ray called pyelography.

The ureters carry urine from the kidney to the bladder for storage. Disorders of the bladder include tumors (malignant or benign), disturbance of bladder control (incontinence), which may be due to another illness such as diabetes or multiple sclerosis, and cystitis. Cystitis, an infection, is also known as painful bladder syndrome and frequency-urgency-dysuria syndrome. About 10% of cystitis patients are men, approximately one-third of whom are over fifty.

FACTS ABOUT THE KIDNEYS

- More than 20 million Americans are affected by kidney and urologic diseases.

- Renal cell carcinoma, the most common form of kidney cancer, usually occurs after the age of 40 and affects twice as many men as women.

- Kidney disease can occur from taking large quantities of painkillers over many years.

- Humans can live in fine health with one kidney. Kidney transplant surgery, however, is not uncommon and is successful in about 80% of all cases.

**THE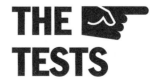
TESTS**

THE URINARY TRACT

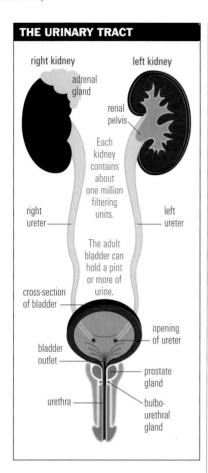

right kidney

left kidney

adrenal gland

renal pelvis

Each kidney contains about one million filtering units.

right ureter

left ureter

The adult bladder can hold a pint or more of urine.

cross-section of bladder

bladder outlet

opening of ureter

prostate gland

urethra

bulbo-urethral gland

including those taken for kidney disease, can flush electrolytes out of the body and cause dehydration.

Magnesium

Along with calcium and phosphorus, magnesium levels in the body can be abnormal in liver disease and kidney failure.

Procedure

Blood is taken from a vein and sent to a lab for analysis.

Results

Magnesium is largely regulated by the kidney. Too little magnesium in the blood is common in liver disease. Too much is usually a sign of overconsumption, such as taking too much antacid. People with kidney failure have too much magnesium because their kidneys cannot get rid of it.

Magnesium is essential in the formation of bones and teeth, for muscle contraction, and for the transmission of nerve impulses. Found in most foods, it is used in many laxatives as well. Taking too much antacid, particularly in cases of kidney disease, can be very harmful, even deadly.

Electrolytes

These compounds must remain in balance in the blood for survival. They are electrically charged minerals naturally found in the body. Four are usually studied: Bicarbonate maintains the body's acid-base balance. Potassium, sodium, and chloride help maintain the body's fluid balance. This test is almost always done at any suspicion of kidney disease, and on every patient who enters the hospital.

Procedure

Blood is drawn from a vein and sent to a lab for analysis.

Results

Testing for their presence is also a test of dehydration, but can be indicative of problems elsewhere. Any diuretic,

Osmolality

Osmolality measures the concentration of dissolved particles in the blood. It evaluates fluid and electrolyte imbalance in the blood and urine. This test is done when the doctor suspects seizures and dehydration.

Procedure

Blood is taken from a vein and sent to a lab for analysis.

Results

Since the kidney is responsible for maintaining these levels, an imbalance may be a sign of kidney disease.

Phosphorus

Most phosphorus in the body is stored in the bones, and helps regulate calcium levels in the body.

Procedure

Blood is taken from a vein and sent to a lab for analysis.

Results

Along with calcium and magnesium, the amount of this substance in the blood can be used to predict kidney failure. Low amounts of calcium and magnesium usually means lots of phosphorus. This condition indicates kidney and liver failure, and thyroid problems too.

> Phosphorus exists outside the body in two forms, yellow and red. Red cannot be absorbed by the body and is nontoxic. Yellow, on the other hand, is readily absorbed and very toxic. It is found in factories, fireworks, and some rat poisons.

Sodium

Sodium is one of the most important minerals in the body. The kidney and brain work together to find a sodium balance. If too much sodium—in the form of table salt—is ingested, the brain will tell the kidney to flush more out of the system.

Procedure

Blood is taken from a vein and sent to a lab for analysis.

Results

Excess sodium building up in the body may be an indicator of kidney failure or malfunction. Diminished sodium in the body is clinically more common than levels which are too high.

Blood Urea Nitrogen (BUN), Creatinine, Creatinine Clearance

These tests are usually done together in a "panel" with the the previous three, and are almost always performed when any kidney trouble is suspected. The kidneys usually filter urea nitrogen and creatinine out of the body.

Procedure

Blood is taken from a vein and sent to a lab for analysis. The creatinine clearance test measures the amount of creatinine in both blood and urine over time, so samples of both are taken over the course of a day.

Results

Presence of too much urea nitrogen or creatinine in the blood is an indication of kidney failure. The creatinine clearance test measures exactly how well the kidney is functioning by checking how much of the waste product is removed, and how fast. This gives doctors important beginning information and can lead to further investigation. Too little BUN in the blood may be an indication of liver problems or of malnutrition.

Urinalysis

This common test evaluates urine based on a number of factors. It can lead to a diagnosis of a huge number of diseases, or merely indicate general health. Because urine is so readily available and any abnormality in the body often causes some abnormality in the urine, this test is universal.

Procedure

The patient urinates into a sample cup which is then sent to a lab for analysis. The urine is then analyzed for color, appearance and odor. The pH (acidity) is taken. A small amount can be cultured to test for bacteria. Some is examined under a microscope, looking for abnormal particles or blood in the urine. Any sediment in the urine can be analyzed and its content determined. Dipsticks, pieces of plastic coated with chemicals that change color in the presence

more tests ⟶

of other chemicals, can be dipped into the urine to test for these chemicals.

Results

Though many tests can be done during a urinalysis, several are always done. The urine is examined visually, and cloudiness or blood indicates a problem. The specific gravity, which measures the volume of particles dissolved in the urine, can alert doctors to kidney problems. A low or high pH can be a sign of kidney failure, infection, diabetes or dehydration. The presence of glucose in the urine indicates diabetes or other kidney problems. Ketones in the urine indicate diabetes or starvation. Nitrite in the urine is a good indication of infection. Protein in the urine usually means the kidney filters have been damaged.

Urine Amino Acid Screen

Usually, only small amounts of amino acids are found in urine. More than a small amount can indicate kidney problems.

Procedure

The patient urinates into a sterile container, which is then sent to a lab for analysis.

Results

An increase of amino acids in urine means that the kidney is not handling them properly, a sign of disease.

Urine Culture

Normal urine is sterile. It contains fluids, salts, and waste products, but is free of bacteria, viruses, and fungi. This test cultures urine to see if bacteria grows, indicating a urinary tract infection. It is usually done during urinalysis.

Procedure

The patient urinates into a sterile container, which is then sent to a lab

for analysis.

Results

Bacteria in the urine is a sign of a urinary tract infection. Antibiotics are usually given to treat the infection.

Urinary tract infections are less common in men than in women, and may be caused by sexual activity or by organisms that have spread from the rectum, bladder or kidneys. They are not uncommon in men who have been hospitalized with a catheter. Careful personal hygiene, drinking plenty of fluids, and regular emptying of the bladder can prevent these infections.

24 Hour Urine (Steroids, calcium and protein)

Since many chemicals in the body fluctuate with food and exercise, looking at one urine sample is often not enough. This tests urine collected over the course of an entire day, every single time the patient urinates.

Procedure

The patient urinates into a sterile container, which is then sent to a lab for analysis. All urine for an entire day is collected for study. The same container is used all day.

Results

The urine is tested for several components. Too much calcium in the urine can be a sign that kidney stones will form or that hormone regulation is damaged. The 24 hour test for protein provides more detailed information about why protein would be in the urine than a standard urinalysis. Uric acid is found in the urine of patients with gout and leukemia, and can contribute to kidney stones as well. Excessive amounts of steroids, produced by the genital organs or other endocrine glands (adrenal glands), can indicate diseases in these organs.

Abdominal X-ray

This test is often the first step in diagnosing abdominal pain. It examines the internal organs of the abdomen, searching for intestinal blockages and tears, tumors and other deposits such as kidney and gallstones (see x-ray under Medical Terms). This test reveals clear pictures of the kidney and bladder, but different, more specialized tests may be required to view the intestines.

Procedure

The patient dons a hospital gown and two x-ray pictures are taken, one lying down and one standing. It is a short and painless test.

Results

Calcium deposits in the kidney and bladder are revealed with this test. If a tumor has blocked the operation of an organ, the backup, not the tumor itself, is visible. Swollen organs are visible, however.

Cystography, Cystourethrogram

Liquid comes to the bladder from the kidney via the ureters, and passes out of the body through the urethra. This test can trace this process with x-rays. The pyelogram may also be conducted for similar purposes. This test is often ordered after an abnormal urinalysis.

Procedure

A catheter is inserted via the urethra into the bladder. The catheter drains any liquid out of the bladder, then injects dye into the bladder. X-rays are then taken.

Results

This test studies the function of the bladder, looking for malfunctions or tumors. If liquid passes back up the ureters toward the kidney, this will be evident on the x-ray. If it leaks out of the bladder, this indicates a tear.

> Incontinence is a term for involuntary urination. Approximately 3 million older Americans suffer with this problem, but men are affected less often than women. It can be caused by infections, stones or tumors. Urinalysis and pyelogram can often detect these problems or other blockages.

Pyelogram

This procedure evaluates kidney function. Kidneys often do not show up well on a standard x-ray, so this procedure, involving a contrast dye, is used.

This test is often ordered after an abnormal urinalysis in order to see the flow of blood in the system more clearly.

Procedure

Before this test is performed, it is common to give the patient a laxative to clear the intestine of material which could interfere with the x-ray. A dye is usually injected intravenously, and the patient then waits for it to spread through the blood to the kidneys. X-rays are taken once, the patient urinates, and then pictures are taken again.

Results

The size and shape of the kidneys are apparent, and any abnormality is evident. Cancer of the kidney can be seen, as can infections and kidney stones. If the dye does not spread properly in the kidneys, this indicates bad blood flow and possible kidney failure. The ureters and bladder are also made visible as the dye passes into them.

Renal Angiogram

Similar to the pyelogram above, this test evaluates kidney function and blood flow. Unlike the pyelogram, dye is injected more directly. This test is often ordered after an abnormal urinalysis and for diagnosis of high blood pressure or renal tumors.

Procedure
First, a local anesthetic is injected into the skin near the femoral artery, a large artery in the leg. A catheter is then inserted into this artery, and it is maneuvered up into the body next to the kidney. The catheter then injects a contrast dye directly into the kidney area, and x-rays are taken.

Results
As with the above test, this diagnoses kidney failure, stones, and cancers. It also diagnoses narrowing of the arteries to the kidneys (blood vessel blockages). It is not taken over a period of time.

Cystoscopy
With this type of endoscopy, the endoscope enters the body through the urethra. This procedure allows the urologist direct examination of the urethra and bladder in order to determine the health of the tissues.

Procedure
The cystoscope is a rigid tube inserted into the penis and up into the bladder. The urethra, the tube through which this scope travels, is anesthetized with an injection beforehand, but the insertion is still painful. A sedative is recommended. The doctor or technician can then look through the tube and perform various tests. Urine, blood or tissue can be sampled. This test provides an advantage over the standard urine test, because it can take urine from either kidney. Dye may also be injected through the scope, and x-rays taken, a procedure called a retrograde pyelogram. This test usually causes a bit of blood in the urine, and urination afterwards is key to avoiding infection.

Results
This test can visually detect problems in the prostate, the kidney and especially the bladder. Tumors or other growths are usually clear. Samples removed can be analyzed for cancer and infection, and x-rays obtained are studied as described above in pyelogram. These x-rays usually show the bladder better than a normal pyelogram. Sometimes, the scope can be used to remove stones.

Cystometry
This test is similar to the one described above, but measures bladder function.

Procedure
The patient first urinates to clear the bladder. A catheter is then inserted into the urethra, and different fluids are inserted and drained out of the bladder. The patient must describe any unusual sensations. The bladder is then filled completely with liquid, measuring the bladder's size and pressure. The fluid may be drained from the bladder and replaced with carbon dioxide for further measurements.

Results
This test measures bladder pressure, sensitivity and other functions. Any abnormalities are reported by the patient or the instruments, and usually lead to further testing. This is an extremely uncomfortable and embarrassing–but safe–test. It is common for the patient to request a sedative before the procedure.

Renin Assay, Plasma
When blood pressure falls, the kidneys release renin, which can be measured in the bloodstream.

Procedure
Blood is taken from a vein and sent to a lab for analysis.

Results
The leakage of this kidney-produced enzyme into the bloodstream is an indication of blood vessel blockage in the kidney area or kidney failure.

More than 260,000 Americans depend upon dialysis because of kidney failure. Dialysis is a mechanical technique which replicates the action of the kidneys, removing waste products from the blood. There are two basic methods. One involves the filtering of blood through an artificial kidney machine outside the body. The other inserts a liquid into the abdomen. The liquid absorbs waste products in the body, and is then drained.

Renogram, Renal Scan

This nuclear scan evaluates blood flow to the kidneys as well as their location and structure. It is the nuclear version of the renal angiography.

Procedure

Several radioisotopes are absorbed specifically by the kidney. One of these is injected into a vein, and it moves to the kidneys. The gamma camera then takes pictures of the kidney area.

Results

This test can show kidney failure, hypertension and cancers. Areas which do not absorb the dye suggest tumors, cysts, and non-function.

For Further Information

National Kidney Foundation
30 East 33rd Street
New York, NY 10016
1-800-622-9010
www.kidney.org

National Association for Continence (NAFC)
P.O. Box 8310
Spartanburg, SC 29305-8310
1-800-BLADDER (1-800-252-3337)
www.nafc.org

American Foundation for Urologic Disease
1128 N. Charles Street
Baltimore, MD 21201
1-800-242-2383
www.afud.org

GALLBLADDER

The gallbladder is a small pear-shaped sac located under the liver. The purpose of the gallbladder is to concentrate and store bile manufactured by the liver before sending it on to the duodenum, where fat digestion occurs. The gallbladder swells between meals as it fills with bile, then expels it into the digestive tract to help food digest. Gallbladder problems are rare in childhood and early adulthood. **Gallstones** are crystals of cholesterol, bile, and pigment that form in the gallbladder. They may obstruct the passage of bile into the intestinal tract, causing inflammation, and symptoms of pain, nausea, and diarrhea or generalized infection. They cause severe pain in the upper abdomen for up to four hours at a time, frequently after a meal.

Although women are twice as likely as men to develop gallstones between the ages of twenty and sixty, the likelihood of developing gallstones increases for both sexes thereafter. Obesity is a major risk factor for gallstone formation, as is crash dieting and prolonged fasting. About 1 million people are diagnosed with gallstones every year, but many carry *silent* stones, which have no symptoms and are usually not problematic.

Gallstones and kidney stones are not related. The most common test for detection of gallstones is the abdominal ultrasound. This is a painless study performed by bouncing sound waves off of the upper quadrant of the abdomen and photographing the image. Gallbladder testing is usually conducted under the supervision of a gastroenterologist, who specializes in disorders of the digestive system.

& PANCREAS

The pancreas is an elongated carrot-shaped gland that lies along the back of the abdomen, behind the stomach. It consists primarily of exocrine tissue which secretes digestive enzymes and hormones into the body. The enzymes break down carbohydrates, fats, proteins, and nucleic acids in the digestive system. The hormones, insulin and glucagon, regulate the level of glucose in the blood.

Because the pancreas is part of both the digestive and the endocrine systems, pancreatic tests may be ordered under the supervision of either a gastroenterologist or an endocrinologist. Diseases of the pancreas include cystic fibrosis (a genetic disorder that predisposes the patient to long term lung infections and prevents the pancreas from producing enzymes essential to the absorption of fat), pancreatitis (which may result from excessive alcohol intake or from viral infection) and pancreatic cancer. **By far the most common pancreatic disorder is diabetes mellitus,** in which the insulin-producing cells in the gland are damaged or destroyed. Insulin helps the sugar from food get into body cells. If the body doesn't make enough insulin, sugar from food cannot get into the cells. Instead, it stays in the blood, elevating blood sugar levels and keeping the body malnourished and tired.

Diabetes, the sixth leading cause of death among those 65 and older, is a major health threat for men. It can cause heart attack, stroke, blindness, impotence, kidney failure, nerve damage, and amputation. Amputation rates are 1.4 to 2.7 times higher in men than in women. Nearly 7.5 million men in the US have Type II diabetes; approximately one-third, or 2.5 million, are not aware that they have it.

Men at risk for Type II diabetes
are over 45
are African-American, American Indian, Latino, or Asian
have a family history of diabetes
are overweight
do not exercise regularly
have low HDL or high triglycerides

Diabetic patients, especially those with poor sugar control, are susceptible to a series of long-term small and large blood vessel complications that can affect every aspect of physical function. Limbs may lose feeling, and eyesight is often affected. Older persons frequently underreport symptoms because they curtail their physical activity to avoid the onset of symptoms, or because their physical function is already impaired by other conditions.

THE 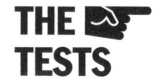
TESTS

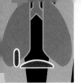
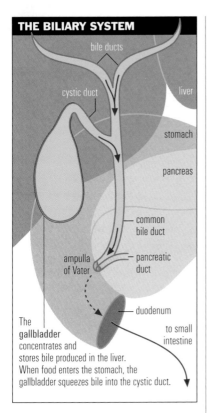

THE BILIARY SYSTEM

bile ducts

cystic duct

liver

stomach

pancreas

common bile duct

ampulla of Vater

pancreatic duct

duodenum

The gallbladder concentrates and stores bile produced in the liver. When food enters the stomach, the gallbladder squeezes bile into the cystic duct.

to small intestine

GALLBLADDER

Endoscopic Retrograde Cholangiopancreatography (ERCP)

For this test see **LIVER** *page 60*

Oral Cholecystogram

If an ultrasound is unable to make a clear diagnosis of pain in the gallbladder, this test will be ordered. The oral cholecystogram utilizes a contrast dye to highlight the gallbladder.

Procedure

In this test, the patient swallows a capsule containing a contrast dye the evening before the test. These capsules can cause side effects, but this is rare. The dye is digested and makes its way into the bile the liver produces. This bile is then stored in the gallbladder about 12 hours after the pill is taken. The x-rays are then taken.

Results

The dye makes the gallbladder stand out on the x-rays. Blockages, inflammations, gallstones, and, rarely, tumors, should all be visible. Cholescintigraphy (Gallbladder Nuclear Scanning, Hepatobiliary scintigraphy, or HIDA scanning) is a procedure that differs from a cholecystogram in that a radionuclide contrast dye is injected in a vein. The dye is again concentrated into the biliary tract and gamma rays emitted from the bile can be detected by a scintillator. This is a help in the diagnosis for gallbladder inflammation or obstruction.

Native Americans have the highest rates of gallstones in the United States. More than half of Native American men have gallstones by age 60.

Percutaneous Transhepatic Cholangiography (PTC)

This test is a different kind of cholangiogram than described under ECRP in the liver section. It is rarely necessary; however, if the dye in the cholecystogram described above does not cause the gallbladder to show up on x-rays, it probably indicates a blockage to the gallbladder. This more invasive test is then performed. Open cholangiograms may be performed during a surgical operation where dye is injected directed into the biliary tracts to make sure that there is no obstruction in this area.

Procedure

The patient is placed on an x-ray table in the radiology department and the abdominal wall or lower chest wall is anesthetized. Using televised fluoroscopic monitoring, a needle is passed through the abdominal wall and into the liver. A biliary branch is located and punctured. When bile is flowing freely into the needle, radiographic dye is injected. The dye passes into the biliary tract. X-rays are then taken. If an obstruction is found, a catheter or stent is left temporarily in the biliary tract to establish drainage and decompression. The patient may feel some discomfort when the needle is introduced, even though the area is anesthetized. This procedure will take approximately one hour. The patient may feel abdominal pain for several hours after the test, and will normally remain under observation for that period.

Results

As above, the dye should make the gall-bladder stand out. Blockages, inflammations, and stones should be visible.

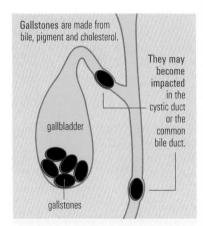

Gallstones are made from bile, pigment and cholesterol.

They may become impacted in the cystic duct or the common bile duct.

gallbladder

gallstones

YOU CAN LIVE WITHOUT A GALLBLADDER

The gallbladder is merely a storage sac which aids in digestion. It is not essential; in fact, some people are born without one. The gallbladder is sometimes removed by a surgical procedure. Each year, more than 500,000 Americans have gallbladder surgery.

A **cholecystectomy** is an operation to remove the gallbladder completely

A **cholecystostomy** opens the gallbladder and removes the stones while leaving the organ itself in place; however, this is rarely done as gallstones may reoccur.

THE TOP 4 WARNING SIGNS OF DIABETES

- Frequent urination.
- Excessive thirst and hunger.
- Family members with diabetes; it often runs in families.
- Sugar binges; diabetes can be detected with blood and urine tests for glucose.

PANCREAS

Amylase

Amylase converts the starch in food into sugar so that it can be used by the body. It is created by the pancreas and salivary glands.

Procedure

Blood is drawn from a vein and sent to a lab for analysis.

Results

If the pancreas or salivary organs are inflamed or damaged, amylase leaks into the bloodstream. Increased presence of this enzyme in the blood indicates these conditions.

C-peptide

This enzyme is in the bloodstream in proportion to insulin, but stays in the body longer, making it a more accurate measure. The blood test for the enzyme is ordered when there is a need to measure insulin.

Procedure

Blood is drawn from a vein and sent to a lab for analysis.

Results

This test is primarily used to monitor insulin in the body, although too much of this enzyme is a sign of renal failure.

Glucose

The body of a diabetic cannot process glucose, the body's blood sugar. This

more tests ☞

blood test measures glucose levels in the body. A variation of the test, called the glucose tolerance test, is ordered on known diabetics. A known (usually large) quantity of glucose is given to the patient to eat, and blood tests are done over time to see how the patient reacts.

Procedure

Blood is drawn from a vein and sent to a lab for analysis. The glucose tolerance test takes both blood and urine samples at half-hour intervals after the meal is eaten.

Results

Too little glucose, hypoglycemia, is a sign of starvation or an overdose of insulin. Symptoms include dizziness and light-headedness. Too much glucose, hyperglycemia, is a strong indication of diabetes.

Insulin allows glucose to be absorbed into the muscle cells and liver, where it can be stored. Hyperglycemia, or high blood sugar, results when not enough insulin is produced to process glucose. Diabetes is defined by the body's inability to produce enough insulin or its ineffective response to insulin. Many diabetics must take insulin shots regularly to process the glucose in their body. If they do not, a coma can result. Hypoglycemia, meaning low blood sugar, results from not eating enough carbohydrates or taking too much insulin or diabetic medication.

Hemoglobin A1C (Glycohemoglobin)

Glucose combines with hemoglobin, a component of blood, to form hemoglobin AlC. This is a storage form of glucose, which stays in the blood long-term and does not fluctuate with meals, as normal glucose would. This test is usually ordered in those who have already had a glucose test which requires further investigation. It monitors the average level of hemoglobin AlC over the ninety days a red blood cell lives.

Diabetes mellitus, the common form of the disease, exists in two types. Type I diabetes usually manifests itself between the ages of 10 and 16. The pancreas suddenly loses its ability to produce insulin. It comes on quickly, and untreated can result in a coma unless the victim injects regularly with insulin. Type II, which is more common, comes on gradually and usually manifests itself after the age of 40.

Diabetes can be controlled. By maintaining blood sugar with insulin injections and/or other medications, a constant weight and healthy lifestyle, it need not greatly alter a person's life. Those who do not monitor the problem, however, can face loss of vision, loss of circulation to the extremities, and pancreatic failure.

Procedure

Blood is drawn from a vein and sent to a lab for analysis.

Results

If high hemoglobin AlC is found as well as high glucose, these factors are a strong indication of diabetes, especially Type II. This test is also used to monitor how well diabetics are controlling their sugar levels with insulin therapy.

Ketones

Ketones, chemical compounds in the blood, exist in high quantities when the body has to burn fat reserves because it is unable to use carbohydrates.

Procedure

Blood is drawn from a vein and sent to a lab for analysis. The patient urinates into a sterile container, which is also sent to a lab.

Results

Both diabetics and people who are

dehydrated or suffering from starvation may exhibit high ketone levels. Ketosis, the accumulation of excessive amounts of Ketones in the body, is usually a medical emergency.

Lipase

The pancreas serves an important function producing digestive enzymes, such as lipase, which digests fats.

Procedure

Blood is drawn from a vein and sent to a lab for analysis.

Results

Elevated levels of this digestive enzyme in the blood occurs when the pancreas is infected or blocked by cysts. This test is less sensitive than the test for amylase, but will detect pancreatic inflammation a longer period of time after the infection occurs.

Pancreatic cancer is one of the most common cancers in the US. It is difficult to diagnose, and has no direct cause, although smoking and fat-heavy diet may be contributors. It is the fourth most common cancer in men, sixth most common in women (1989). Eighty percent of cases occur in people over 50.

Sweat Test

Patients with cystic fibrosis have high levels of several minerals in their sweat. This disease, which patients are born with, can be treated if detected early.

Procedure

The area to be tested is cleaned and dried. A drug which induces sweat is dropped onto the skin. An electrode is placed on top of the skin, and another on a nearby patch of skin. Low voltage current run between them allows the drug to seep in and sweating begins. The skin is cleaned and dried again, and a piece of absorbent paper is placed on the skin. It absorbs sweat for up to an hour.

Results

The sweat can be tested for the presence of minerals which indicate cystic fibrosis.

Just as diabetes prevents the pancreas from secreting hormones, cystic fibrosis prevents it from secreting the enzymes necessary for digestion of fats, causing malnutrition. This genetic disorder, which also causes lung damage and infections, is treated with antibiotics and digestive supplements. Untreated, it can be fatal. Cystic fibrosis is the most common inherited disease for Caucasians.

For Further Information

GALLBLADDER

National Digestive Diseases
Information Clearinghouse
2 Information Way
Bethesda, MD 20892-3570
www.nddk.nih.gov/health/digest/
pubs/gallstns

American Gastrointestinal
Association
www.gastro.org/gallstones.html

American Society for
Gastrointestinal Endoscopy (ASGE)
www.asge.org

PANCREAS

The National Pancreas Foundation
P.O. Box 600590
Newtonville, MA 02460
1-877-NPF-FUND (1-877-673-3863)
www.pancreasfoundation.org/

Pancreas.org: An Informational Site
www.pancreas.org

National Institute of Diabetes and
Digestive and Kidney Diseases
Diabetes Prevention Program
www.preventdiabetes.com.

80

UPPER GI

The stomach is an organ of the digestive system, connected to the esophagus (swallowing tube) above and the duodenum (the first part of the small intestine) below. **As any man who has let his belt out a notch after a big meal can attest, the stomach is elastic and expands when food is eaten.** In an adult, the average stomach capacity is about 1.5 quarts (or three pints). Because the stomach is also a reservoir, disorders which occur in the process of emptying the contents include tumors, gastritis (inflammation of the stomach lining), and peptic ulcers, the most common serious stomach ailment.

Ulcers occur when stomach acid and other digestive juices attack and break down the stomach or intestinal lining,

and can result from stress, injury or infection. Ulcers are more common after the age of 60. The incidence of **gastric ulcers** is about equal in men and women, but more men than women suffer from **duodenal ulcers.**

THE TOP 5 SIGNS OF STOMACH ULCERS

- Gnawing pain, particularly when the stomach is empty.

- Loss of appetite.

- Excessive gas or vomiting. Vomiting blood or blood in the stool usually means the ulcer is bleeding, a medical emergency.)

- Feeling bloated.

- Weight loss.

The esophagus is the tube which carries food from the mouth to the stomach. Esophagitis is the inflammation of the esophagus — commonly causing the symptom of **heartburn.** The small intestine is about 21 feet long and it is here that food absorption occurs. Problems with the stomach, esophagus, and small intestine are frequently treated by a gastroenterologist.

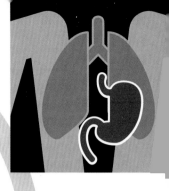

A BITE'S PROGRESS: PART ONE

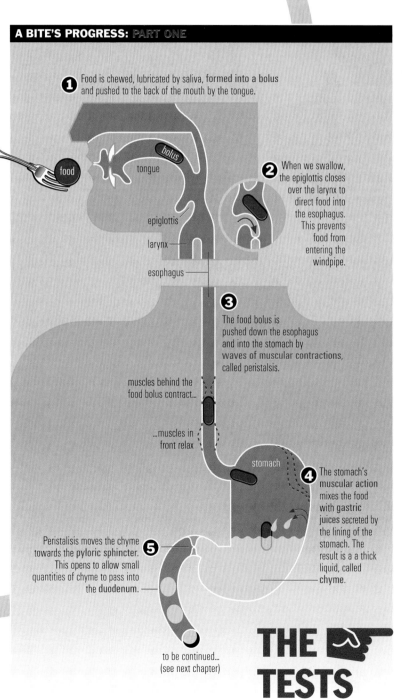

1 Food is chewed, lubricated by saliva, formed into a bolus and pushed to the back of the mouth by the tongue.

bolus

food

tongue

epiglottis

larynx

esophagus

2 When we swallow, the epiglottis closes over the larynx to direct food into the esophagus. This prevents food from entering the windpipe.

3 The food bolus is pushed down the esophagus and into the stomach by waves of muscular contractions, called peristalsis.

muscles behind the food bolus contract...

...muscles in front relax

stomach

4 The stomach's muscular action mixes the food with gastric juices secreted by the lining of the stomach. The result is a a thick liquid, called chyme.

5 Peristalisis moves the chyme towards the pyloric sphincter. This opens to allow small quantities of chyme to pass into the duodenum.

to be continued...
(see next chapter)

THE 👉 TESTS

ANATOMY OF AN ULCER

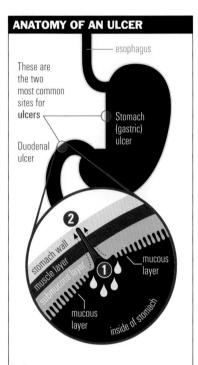

esophagus

These are the two most common sites for ulcers

Stomach (gastric) ulcer

Duodenal ulcer

stomach wall
muscle layer
submucous layer

mucous layer

mucous layer

inside of stomach

1 The stomach's protective layer of mucous is broken down by increased acid secretion.

2 In time, the ulcer may penetrate all three of the stomach's layers, including the outer wall. This can cause peritonitis.

Gastrin Blood Test

Gastrin is a hormone which stimulates acid secretion and can be measured by a blood test.

Procedure

Blood is drawn from a vein and sent to a lab for analysis. Sometimes injections of substances which stimulate gastrin production are given before the blood sample is taken. This helps determine the cause of high gastrin levels.

Results

Excessive gastrin may indicate tumors (usually in the pancreas). This test is useful in patients with ulcer disease.

Men and women develop ulcers equally; up to 10 percent of the population will have an ulcer at some point in their lives. Smoking, drinking alcohol or caffeine, and taking aspirin can irritate an ulcer.

Approximately 20 million Americans will suffer with an ulcer in their lifetimes

Fecal Occult Blood Test

This test examines the patient's stool for the presence of hidden (or occult) blood.

Procedure

A small sample of stool is obtained by the patient either at home or in the doctor's office for analysis in the laboratory.

Results

If the test indicates that there is blood present in the stool, it does not necessarily indicate cancer. A number of non-cancerous bleeding conditions, such as hemorrhoids or ulcers, may exist. This is a standard preventive or screening test often requested by doctors in the course of periodic check-ups and should not be regarded with concern.

Upper GI Series or Barium Swallow

Barium is an important element in x-ray procedures. It coats the interior of the digestive system and shows up well on x-ray film. In particular, tumors and ulcers become more apparent on x-rays using barium.

Procedure

The patient first drinks about 4 ounces of the chalky barium liquid, which is often flavored to make it more palatable. The barium coats the esophagus, stomach and small intestine. X-rays are taken as it does so and after it has had time to settle. These can be taken both sitting up and lying down. It spreads into the stomach for x-ray in about half an hour, but can take 4 hours to spread to the small intestine.

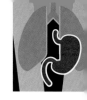

The barium may cause constipation. Although the "barium cocktail" is distasteful to most patients, it is a safe and important diagnostic tool.

Results

Tumors and ulcers should stand out in the esophagus and stomach due to the outlining effect of the barium. If tumors are detected in a barium swallow procedure, a biopsy is usually required for further analysis. The extent of damage from reflux, the bubbling of stomach juices up into the esophagus, can be seen as well.

Esophageal cancer may present difficulty in swallowing. Tumorous obstructions can completely prohibit food from getting to the stomach. This cancer is more common in those over 50.

Esophagogastroduodenoscopy (EGD) or Gastroscopy or Upper GI Endoscopy

This endoscopy is often ordered when ulcers, severe heartburn, or other upper GI (gastrointestinal) disorders are present or suspected. Symptoms of these may include vomiting, especially with blood, and upper abdominal pain, or pain associated with eating and swallowing.

Procedure

The patient must usually fast for several hours beforehand to empty the stomach of all contents. The throat is anesthetized with a spray, and a sedative is given so the patient relaxes. The flexible endoscope is inserted through the mouth, down the esophagus and into the stomach and duodenum (first part of the small intestine). The interior of these organs can be examined and tests can be performed using the endoscope (see endoscopy in Medical Terms). This procedure will require 20 to 30 minutes to perform.

The duodenum refers to the first 10 inches or so of the small intestine. The pyloric sphincter, a muscle ring, connects the stomach to the duodenum and allows food to pass through at regular intervals. Ducts from the pancreas, liver and gallbladder feed bile and enzymes into the duodenum to digest food.

Results

Ulcers are the most common problem discovered during this test. They can be seen through the endoscope. Inflammation or cancers of the stomach and of the esophagus can be seen, and biopsied. This is an excellent method of finding the cause of bleeding in this part of the body. The endoscope may irritate the throat lining and leave the patient with a mild sore throat for a day or so. Because patients may require a sedative before this test, check before arriving to see if you need someone to give you a ride home.

Gastric Analysis

This test measures the amount and composition of juices in the stomach. The amount and quality of acid can help find the cause of ulcer disease or assess treatment.

Procedure

The test begins with the patient fasting up to eight hours before the test, to ensure that the stomach will be completely empty. A narrow, flexible tube is inserted through the nose and down into the stomach. Every fifteen minutes for one hour, the doctor or technician withdraws a sample of stomach juice from the tube. Then the patient is injected with a chemical that will cause the stomach to produce acid. Generally, four more samples are collected every fifteen minutes.

more tests ▷

Results

The samples are analyzed and compared for their acid content. If the injected chemical has no effect on acid production in the stomach, this may indicate gastritis, gastric ulcer, or cancer. Increased acid in the stomach is associated with ulcers, tumors, and endocrine disease.

Over 60 million Americans experience acid indigestion (also called Gastroesophageal Reflux Disease or GERD) at least once a month.

Stomach cancer can be misdiagnosed as indigestion, and is more prevalent in those over 50. Some signs of stomach cancer: persistent feeling of fullness, pain before or after meals, change in digestion habits.

Approximately 24,000 Americans are diagnosed with cancer of the stomach each year.

Helicobacter Pylori Tests

This microbe, which is recognized as contributing to gastric diseases such as duodenal ulcers, gastritis, and gastric carcinoma, can be detected by several methods, depending upon diagnostic needs.

Procedures

The helicobacter pylori bacteria is found in the mucus layer that lines the stomach and can be identified by a cultured specimen, a gastric mucosal biopsy, a blood test, or a breath test.

A biopsy or mucus specimen for culturing may be obtained by an esophagogastroduodenoscopy (EGD), as described above. The specimen should be transported to the lab within thirty minutes of collection. Analysis of blood drawn from a vein, however, is an equally accurate and simpler procedure. The breath test requires the patient to swallow a dose of radioactive C or nonradioactive C urea.

Results

A biopsy or culture will be tested for heliobacter pylori or for antibodies. Similarly, blood can be analyzed for the presence of these antibodies. The breath test is based on the ability of helicobacter pylori to break down urea into carbon dioxide and ammonia. The CO_2 concentration will reveal the presence of the microbe.

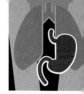

For Further Information:

National Digestive Diseases
Information Clearinghouse
2 Information Way
Bethesda, MD 20892-3570
www.niddk.nih.gov/health/digest/
pubs/diagtest/

Crohn' s & Colitis Foundation of
America, Inc.
386 Park Avenue South, 17th Floor
New York, NY 10016-8804
1-800-932-2423

American Gastrointestinal
Association
www.gastro.org

International Foundation for
Functional Gastrointestinal
Disorders (IFFGD)
P.O. Box 117864
Milwaukee, WI 53217
1-888-964-2001

The American College of
Gastroenterology (ACG)
1-800-978-7666
www.acg.gi.org/patientinfo/

Society of American Gastrointestinal
Endoscopic Surgeons (SAGES)
www.medscape.com/SAGES/
Patientinformation/pi.09.html

LOWER GI

The colon is a segmented tube approximately four and a half feet long that forms the major portion of the large intestine. It has four sections: ascending, transverse, descending, and sigmoid colon. Rhythmic contractions of the muscles along the colon push the intestinal contents through the colon to the rectum. Food has been completely digested before it enters the colon, where the primary function is to absorb water before waste leaves the body. Disorders of the colon and lower gastrointestinal system include diverticular disease, ulcerative colitis, and tumors. Diverticulosis, the formation of small sacs in the intestine which protrude from its walls, is present in half of the US population by the age of 80. This condition is permanent, and when these small sacs become inflamed (diverticulitis) the patient requires antibiotic treatment. Ulcerative colitis is an inflammation of the lining of the colon, causing bloody stool. (There are several causes of inflammation. Ulcerative colitis is only one cause.) It can lead to an increased risk of cancer, but can be treated with steroid-type drugs. Doctors who specialize in the health of the lower gastrointestinal tract are called gastroenterologists.

Colorectal cancer is one of the most common cancers. After lung cancer, it is the leading cause of cancer deaths. Incidence increases with age, beginning at about age 40. It is a common misconception that colon cancer is a disease that primarily strikes men. An equal number of men and women die from colon cancer each year. Approximately 130,000 Americans were diagnosed with the disease in 1998, half of them men. **More than 55,000 people were diagnosed too late for effective treatment and died.** Unfortunately only 20% of American adults are regularly tested for colorectal cancer.

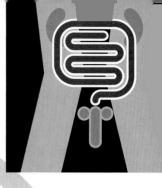

A BITE'S PROGRESS: PART TWO

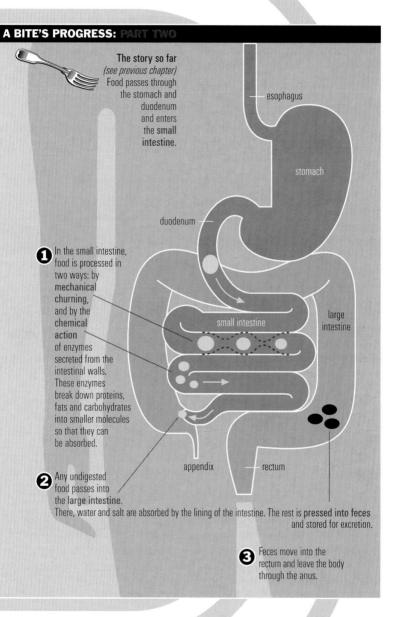

The story so far
(see previous chapter)
Food passes through
the stomach and
duodenum
and enters
the small
intestine.

esophagus

stomach

duodenum

❶ In the small intestine,
food is processed in
two ways: by
**mechanical
churning,**
and by the
**chemical
action**
of enzymes
secreted from the
intestinal walls.
These enzymes
break down proteins,
fats and carbohydrates
into smaller molecules
so that they can
be absorbed.

small intestine

large
intestine

❷ Any undigested
food passes into
the large intestine.
There, water and salt are absorbed by the lining of the intestine. The rest is **pressed into feces**
and stored for excretion.

appendix

rectum

❸ Feces move into the
rectum and leave the body
through the anus.

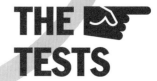

THE
TESTS

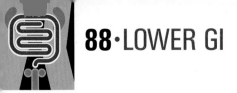

Routine Stool Lab Tests (Occult Blood, Stool and Rectal Cultures)

Along with blood and urine, the contents of stool can provide clues to a variety of diagnoses. Like blood and urine, it is readily available and can be subjected to a battery of tests. This is one of the most common and most important tests of the lower gastrointestinal tract.

Stool is formed through the interworkings of the intestines and the liver. Normal stool is made up of water, minerals, bile, food and bacteria.

Procedure

A stool sample provided by the patient is studied for overall appearance and then evaluated for fat content, in order to diagnose potential problems in the intestinal tract. Cultures can be conducted on stool samples to detect certain harmful bacteria, which can then be treated. Stool is also examined for parasites and blood. The presence of blood may be the first sign of a tumor, and is therefore an important diagnostic indicator. The patient should avoid red meat for two days prior to this test to avoid false positive results. Bleeding may also be caused by ASA or Motrin or other non-steroidal anti-inflammatory medications.

Results

Abnormalities in the consistency, content, odor and color of stool may reflect disease anywhere along the path food travels from top to bottom. Stool naturally contains a lot of bacteria. Some, however, are indications of abnormalities or poisons in the intestine, and these can be identified in the test. Blood in the stool, usually not evident to the naked eye, is often an indication of cancer, colitis, ulcer formation, hemorrhoids or inflammation. Stool is also examined for para-

sites or eggs. If blood is in the stool, this test leads to others, such as Sigmoidoscopy, Barium enema or Colonoscopy.

Proctosigmoidoscopy or Sigmoidoscopy

The purpose of this test is to see the lining of the sigmoid colon. The last 10 inches of the gastrointestinal tract are often those most plagued by disease. Frequent problems include bleeding, hemorrhoids and pain. This endoscopy examines only the lowest part of the intestinal tract. For patients over the age of 50, this test is often a preventive screening test for cancer.

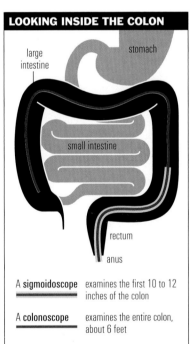

LOOKING INSIDE THE COLON

large intestine

stomach

small intestine

rectum

anus

A **sigmoidoscope** examines the first 10 to 12 inches of the colon

A **colonoscope** examines the entire colon, about 6 feet

Procedure

The patient is given oral laxatives or an enema just before the test to clear the colon. The patient then lies on an examination table, knees up to chest, as the doctor inserts the lubricated proctosigmoidoscope (a short, rigid tube) or sigmoidoscope (a 10" to 12" tube – sometimes rigid and sometimes flexible – about the size of an index finger) into the rectum. These devices differ from the colonoscope, which is a 42" to 72" flexible tube containing fiber optics. Material may be taken for biopsy as well.

Results

The doctor can see directly what may be causing the problems the patient is having. These diagnoses include polyps, colitis and cancer. Biopsy material can be investigated by a lab, and some growths can be removed. If something suspect is discovered, a Colonoscopy may be ordered.

THE TOP 3 REASONS TO HAVE A SIGMOIDOSCOPY

- It has been shown to locate 80% of all polyps in the colon.

- The test is associated with a 59% to 80% reduction in risk of death from cancer in the part of the colon examined.

- Periodic tests reduce anxiety about normal gastric distress.

Colonoscopy

In this test, the endoscope enters the colon through the rectum and moves up through it, examining for cancer, colitis, and polyps. The colonoscope which is used during the test is a flexible tube about as thick as an index finger which is 42" to 72" long. It contains fiber optics which light the interior of the colon for better visibility and can allow the technician to obtain computer visualizations of the colon.

Procedure

The patient takes a heavy laxative the night before the test, and cannot eat much of the day before to clear the colon completely. Sometimes additional enemas are needed. The patient lies on his left side on an examination table with knees drawn up. The doctor then lubricates and

inserts the colonoscope into the rectum. This is uncomfortable but not usually painful. Air is sometimes passed through the scope to inflate the bowel, allowing the scope to penetrate further. This causes a cramping feeling of fullness in the patient. The images transmitted from the end of the scope appear on a screen, which the doctor studies as the scope is removed. A sedative is often given to relax the patient both physically and mentally before the test. The patient may need to have a friend drive home after the test.

Results

The doctor can see any abnormalities inside the colon during this test. These include tumors, polyps, colitis and diverticular disease. Fluid samples or biopsy material gathered by the colonoscope may be analyzed for similar conditions.

Barium Enema or Air Contrast Enema

This type of x-ray is used to obtain images of the colon indirectly with x-ray films. Barium, which absorbs x-rays, lines the colon and x-rays are taken.

Each year, about 131,000 people are diagnosed with colon cancer. The cancer begins with polyps, benign, small growths on the inside of the colon. 90% of colon cancer can be cured if these polyps are removed before the cancer spreads to the lymph nodes, so early detection is key.

Procedure

The patient's colon is first cleared out, either with a laxative or by fasting, or, if needed, enemas. After a plain x-ray of the colon is taken first, the barium enema is inserted into the patient's rectum. A balloon on the enema inflates to hold it inside the

more tests ▶

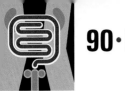
rectum, and barium begins to flow into the colon. As it is distributed through the colon, additional x-ray pictures are taken. Sometimes, air is introduced through the enema as well, causing the barium to coat the colon thinly for clearer pictures. This is called an air contrast enema. The presence of barium or air produces a feeling of fullness and makes the patient feel the need to defecate immediately. It is not unusual for patients to expel some of the liquid. The patient should not feel embarrassed if this occurs. Barium will color the patient's stool light for several days, as it is expelled. The barium is safe and is not absorbed in the body.

Results

The barium makes polyps, tumors, and diverticular disease much more visible than the normal x-ray would. These problems can then be identified and treated.

Diet, body weight and physical activity all contribute to a healthy colon. A diet high in vegetables, fruits and grains, and low in animal fat will help reduce the risk. Calcium may also have a risk-reducing effect.

CT Colonoscopy

In 1996, researchers at the Bowman Gray School of Medicine in Winston-Salem, N.C. developed a new x-ray scanning procedure that is less expensive, more comfortable, and less time-consuming than barium enemas or colonoscopy. Clinical trials are under way to determine whether this technique is effective. Until these studies are completed, this procedure should not be considered a standard of care.

Procedure

After the patient has had cleansing enemas or has fasted, air is inserted into the colon. A helical CT scanner passing painlessly over the patient requires less than two minutes to gather two-dimensional images that can be reconstructed to show doctors and technicians views of the colon that are sliced vertically, horizontally, and in cross-section.

Results

The images from the CT scan reveal all polyps that are larger than one centimeter in size and most other smaller polyps. Polyps larger than one centimeter have a higher likelihood of becoming cancerous. A three-dimensional version of this same technology, known as a virtual colonoscopy, is under development. This would provide views as though a camera were travelling through the colon.

Laparoscopy

This type of endoscopy is used to examine unexplained abdominal pain. The procedure allows the doctor to see the outer surface of all the abdominal organs.

Procedure

The lower abdomen is cleaned and sterilized, and general anesthesia is administered. A small incision is made in the skin and the laparoscope slipped inside. The scope is then used to observe and test the internal organs as during any endoscopy. The scope will be used to fill the abdominal cavity with air, making viewing easier.

Results

From this perspective, doctors can detect cancers and liver disease. It lets them have direct observation of these organs. Any fluid collected or biopsy material can also be analyzed.

Carcinoembryonic Antigen Blood Test (CEA)

Seventy percent of patients with

colon cancer have an elevated level of this antigen in their blood.

Procedure
Blood is drawn from a vein and sent to a lab for analysis.

Results
Although this is helpful in following known cases of colon cancer, it is not a good screening test. The antigen is also elevated in cases of cancers elsewhere in the body and in the blood of smokers. It is often used to monitor therapy and detect a recurrence of cancer as well.

Rectal Digital Examination
Although this test is part of every routine physical examination, it is worth explaining because many men are embarrassed or discomforted by this procedure. The importance of the exam is that it is a quick and simple way for a physician to observe any irregularities in the rectal area.

Procedure
The patient is asked to remove or lower his pants and underwear and lie on his side on an examination table. He may wish to put on a hospital gown, although this is not necessary. The doctor wears sterile latex gloves, and, using one finger, he probes and touches the anal area and the entrance to the rectum. The stimulation from the insertion of the doctor's finger may cause some men to experience an erection. However, this is quite normal and not cause for alarm.

Results
This rectal examination may allow the doctor to detect enlargement or hardening of the prostate gland. The doctor may also note the presence of hemorrhoidal tissues or scarring in the rectal area. In addition, any polyps or growths detected in the rectum might require removal or biopsy for further diagnosis

For Further Information

National Cancer Information Service
9000 Rockville Pike
Bethesda, MD 20892
301-496-4000

Agency for Health Care Policy and Research Publications Clearinghouse
P.O. Box 8547
Silver Spring, MD 20907
1-800-358-9295
www.ahcpr.gov/

National Digestive Diseases Information Clearinghouse
2 Information Way
Bethesda, MD 20892-3570
www.niddk.nih.gov/health/digest/pubs/diagtest/

American Gastrointestinal Association
www.gastro.org/

The American College of Gastroenterology (ACG)
1-800-978-7666
www.acg.gi.org/patientinfo/

Society of American Gastrointestinal Endoscopic Surgeons (SAGES)
www.medscape.com/SAGES/Patientinformation/pi.09.html

REPRODUCTIVE SYSTEM

If men in general are resistant to medical testing (and they are), they are especially resistant to testing of their reproductive systems. After all, this is an assault on their manhood—literally. The penis, testicles and surrounding organs make up the male genitalia. The testicles produce sperm and the male hormone testosterone. The main health risks to the male reproductive system are sexually transmitted diseases (STD) and cancer.

The prostate gland is a solid, walnut-shaped organ surrounding the base of the urethra inside the body below the bladder. The prostate grows through puberty, stops, and then begins to grow again around age 40. As it grows, it may constrict urinary flow. **Benign prostatic hypertrophy (aka BPH, or an enlarged prostate) is common in men over the age of 50.** This usually manifests itself in difficulty in urination or continuing to feel full after urination. Although cancer of the testicles is relatively rare, **prostate cancer is the second most common cause of death from cancer in men of all ages,** killing over 40,000 men each year. It is the most common cause of death from cancer in men over 75 years old, but is rarely found in men younger than 40 years of age. **Prostate cancer does not strike all ethnic groups equally;** African-American men have the highest prostate cancer rate of any racial or ethnic group in the country.

Early identification of prostate cancer is now possible by annual screening of men over 50. (Because of their greater susceptibility to prostate cancer, it is recommended that African-American men and those with a family history of prostate cancer begin annual screening earlier, at age 40.) This screening involves a digital rectal examination (DRE) and a PSA (prostate specific antigen) blood test. Additionally, a transrectal prostate ultrasound and biopsy may be performed to evaluate suspicious areas.

TO TEST OR NOT TO TEST?

Whether early detection or screening for prostate cancer really makes a difference is still a source of debate among experts. The complete and final answer will require several years of careful studies. However, the preliminary evidence supports prostate checks for early detection of prostate cancer in most American men over 50 years of age. Here are some data:

- Between 1977 and 1981, 54% of all men diagnosed with prostate cancer in the US had prostate cancers confined to the prostate gland, and therefore potentially curable. 46% of men had more advanced and incurable disease in this group.

- Between 1986 and 1992, 67% of Caucasian American men and 62% of African-American men diagnosed with prostate cancer had localized disease and were potentially curable when diagnosed.

- The overall 5 year survival rate for patients diagnosed with prostate cancer in 1985-1986 was only 59%

- The overall 5 year survival rate for patients diagnosed with prostate cancer in 1986 through 1992 was 89% for Caucasian Americans and 73% for African Americans.

THE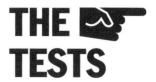
TESTS

Prostate Specific Antigen (PSA)

PSA is normally found in all men; however, PSA levels in the blood are elevated in those who have developed prostate cancer.

Procedure

Blood is drawn and sent to the lab. No fasting or fluid restriction is required.

Results

Men with prostate cancer have elevated PSA levels in their blood. Those who have already been diagnosed with prostate cancer may undergo regular PSA testing to monitor the progress of the disease and/or the effectiveness of therapy. It is important to note that elevated PSA levels are not necessarily indicative of prostate cancer. BPH (benign prostatic hypertrophy) and prostatitis (an infection of the prostate) will also generate elevated PSA levels in the blood.

There is considerable disagreement in the medical community over the use of PSA blood tests and the treatment of prostate cancer in older men. While reputable specialists argue that PSA tests will reveal cancerous cells in the prostate, this type of cancer is so slow-growing that most men over 65 will die of other causes before this cancer can be fatal. If surgery is undertaken, it leaves a substantial number of men impotent and incontinent. Doctors in favor of PSA testing and prostate cancer treatment point out that more than 34,000 men die from prostate cancer each year. Each case is different, and you must discuss the pros and cons of this testing with your doctor.

Scrotal/Prostate Ultrasound

These types of ultrasound are useful in detecting disorders of the prostate and testicles, and can identify even non-palpable cancers.

Procedure

The patient is first given an enema. For a prostate ultrasound, the doctor examines the rectum and inserts the ultrasound probe. The probe gives off sound waves into the prostate. The sound waves which are bounced back appear on the screen, giving a picture of the area. For a testicular ultrasound, a jelly is spread on the scrotum and the testicles are visualized.

Results

Prostate ultrasound is a great aid in the specific diagnosis of prostate cancer. Testicular ultrasound detects tumors of the testicles.

Cystoscopy

For this test see **KIDNEYS** *page 72*

Infertility Testing/Semen Analysis

The top cause of male infertility is failure to produce enough healthy sperm. Sperm may be defective, blocked from leaving the body, or not produced in enough quantity by the testicles. Many semen tests are available to study male fertility. All require a sample.

Procedure

The patient provides a fresh sample of semen at a testing facility.

Results

Semen analysis is the first test done for male infertility. It can reveal abnormal sperm, low sperm count and "lazy" sperm, which lack the ability to swim effectively. In addition, a blockage may be preventing sperm from leaving the body. Blockages are sometimes due to STDs such as gonorrhea. As many as one in six couples may have fertility problems.

AIDS Blood Serology

AIDS is the most serious STD. It

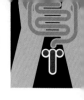

acts by suppressing the immune system, magnifying the impact of otherwise mild, treatable illnesses. Those at most risk are sexually active homosexual and bisexual men, women with multiple partners, intravenous drug users, persons receiving blood tainted with HIV (the virus that causes AIDS), and infants exposed to the disease while in utero. AIDS develops from the HIV virus in one to five percent of those infected each year. A number of different tests exist for the disease, and testing positive with one test does not necessarily mean that AIDS is present. Positive results from one type of test are confirmed with an alternative diagnostic technique. If one test is positive and another negative, the patient should retest in three to six months. Home HIV tests are now available, but no test is yet 100 percent conclusive.

Procedure

Blood is drawn from a vein and sent to a lab for analysis.

Results

This blood test detects the HIV antibodies which lead to the AIDS virus. A positive test means that the patient has the human immunodeficiency virus, which can develop into full-blown AIDS

There is no cure for AIDS and no vaccine at present. Various drugs and drug combinations can treat the symptoms of AIDS effectively and prevent HIV from becoming AIDS, at least for a time. HIV is found in many bodily fluids, but it has only been proven to be transmitted through blood and semen. AIDS is not spread through touching, breathing the air an infected person has breathed, or by sharing utensils. Ten percent of AIDS cases occur in people over the age of 50. Although they could have been infected at a younger age, few people in this group ever are tested. Sometimes the disease is mistaken for other signs of aging.

Impotence is rarely psychological. The most common causes are vascular problems, nerve damage, low testosterone and drug side effects.

Herpes Test

Herpes simplex virus (HSV) has two types. Type 1 produces cold sores and fever blisters, generally in the mouth area. HSV Type 2 is a sexually transmitted viral infection whose first manifestation is usually sores. Genital herpes begins as red spots on the penis which then grow, rupture, and ooze. Sores can also appear on and in the mouth, or on other parts of the body. The lesions usually turn up about a week after sex with an infected person, and take 10 to 21 days to heal. Even after the abscesses subside, the person remains infected, and outbreaks of the sores may flare up again in the future. Although forty percent of those affected never have a second attack, recurrences most often take place when the body is run down. Herpes is virulent and extremely contagious when the sores are present. Though diagnosed largely by sight, a fluid sample can be taken from a sore and tested, identifying this STD for monitoring.

Procedure

A swab is used to remove fluid from a suspected herpes lesion. The fluid is then examined under a microscope and cultured. Blood can also be taken from a vein and sent to a lab for analysis.

Results

If the infection grows in the culture, the patient is infected. Herpes is an infection that can become chronic. There is no known cure, although medications to treat the symptoms are quite effective.

more tests ▶

Chlamydia is the most common STD in the U.S., with more than 900,000 cases reported annually. There are more than 600,000 new cases of Gonorrhea diagnosed each year.

Gonorrhea, Chlamydia Blood Tests

Chlamydia is the most frequently occurring STD in the US. The infection begins with unusual discharge from the penis, and often causes pain in urination. Eventually it can cause infertility in both sexes. In cases of chlamydia the symptoms are often mild or misattributed.

About 35% of those who have chlamydia also have gonorrhea. It is a similar infection, both causing cloudy discharge or pain in urination, as well as an urge to urinate often. Gonorrhea can also lead to infertility. It primarily infects the genitals, but can spread as well. It can be transmitted through oral, anal or vaginal sex.

Procedure

A culture is usually taken by swabbing the urethra, collecting some of the infected material present. In the case of gonorrhea, the infection may be visible under a microscope. Blood may also be drawn from a vein and sent to a lab for analysis.

Results

The most reliable test is a culture test in which urethal discharge is cultivated to see if it will grow the bacteria of these infections. If either grows, the patient is infected. Both gonococcal and chlemyolial infections are now treated with antimicrobial drugs such as doxycycline or azithromycin, because many strains of STD have become resistant to penicillin. Patients with a positive diagnosis should advise their sexual partners to be tested. Many states require this test before a marriage license is issued.

Syphilis Blood Test

Syphilis was once so common in Europe it was deemed an epidemic. Now it is quite rare, but it is still an active STD. It can be spread by transfusion or by direct sexual contact.

Procedure

Blood is drawn from a vein and sent to a lab for analysis.

Results

The test looks for antibodies produced in response to treponema pallidum, the spiral- shaped bacterium that causes syphilis. Blood can also be examined under a microscope to look for the syphilis bacteria. Penicillin is a cure for syphilis. Many states require this test before a marriage license is granted.

Testicular Self-exam

Because testicular cancer often produces no symptoms, many doctors recommend monthly self-exams.

Procedure

The best time to examine your testicles is during or right after a warm bath or shower. The heat causes the skin of the scrotum to soften and relax. And, soapy skin may make it even easier to feel any lumps underneath. Examine each testicle separately with both hands by rolling the testicle between the thumbs and fingers. You'll feel a cord-like structure (the epididymis which stores and transports sperm) on the top and back of the testicle. Gently separate this tube from the testicle with your fingers to examine the testicle itself. Feel for any swelling, lumps or any change in the size, shape or consistency of the testes.

Results

Although most are not cancer, any lumps or other symptoms should be checked by a physician immediately.

ABOUT CANCER

- Presently, it is estimated that for every 8 men diagnosed with prostate cancer, only one will die of the disease.

- Prostate cancers spreads by extending into the seminal vesicles, bladder, and rarely into the peritoneal cavity. Prostate cancers typically metastasize to the lymph nodes, bones, lungs and liver. Prostate cancers are classified or staged based on their aggressiveness and the degree that they are different from the surrounding prostate tissue.

- Most prostate cancers are staged using the Whitmore-Jewett system or TNM (international classification system):

  A or T1 Tumor not palpable (able to be felt) but detectable in microscopic biopsy

  B or T2 Palpable tumor confined to prostate

  C or T3 Extension of tumor beyond prostate with no distant metastasis

  D or N1 Cancer has spread to regional
  and M1   lymph nodes

- Both PSA testing and treatment of prostate cancer are areas of disagreement within in the medical community, and a frank discussion of the pros and cons with your doctor is appropriate. Even if prostate cancer is detected, your physician may recommend that no action be taken. Surgery and radiation therapies have undesirable side effects whose serious draw-backs may outweigh the benefits of aggres-sively treating a slow-growing cancer, espe-cially in a man of advanced age. A majority of prostate cancers will not leave the prostate, but doctors are unsure how to pre-dict which ones will move on and become more dangerous.

- Cancers of the penis or testicles are quite rare. Testicular cancer is most common in males under the age of 40, almost never in the elderly.

For Further Information

National Cancer Institute
1-800-422-6237
http://cancernet.nci.nih.gov/clinpdq/
pif/Prostate_cancer_Patient.html

Prostate Cancer Research Institute
www.prostatepointers.org/
strum

American Academy of Family
Physicians
11400 Tomahawk Creek
Parkway, Leawood, KS 66211-2672.
1-800-274-2237 or (913) 906-6000
www.aafp.org

Reducing Your Risk of Prostate
Cancer
American Institute for Cancer
Research
1759 R Street, NW
Washington, DC 20069
1-800-842-4224

Prostate Cancer Information Center
www.findinfo.com/

National Centers for Disease Control
and Prevention
www.cdc.gov

National STD Hotline
1-800-227-8922

National AIDS Hotline
1-800-342-2437

National Institute on Aging
Information Center
1-800-222-2225

more tests ☞

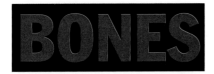

The human skeleton is comprised of bones—long, short, flat, round, irregular—which provide a rigid framework for the surrounding muscles and protect the essential organs in the skull and chest cavity. Although the more than 200 bones in the body vary widely in size and shape, all are subject to the same diseases—fractures, tumors, congenital defects, mineral loss, and infections (osteomyelitis). Broken bones due to accident or injury are a common occurrence in childhood. The most common bone diseases which arise with increasing frequency later in life include bone cancer and osteoporosis.

Osteoporosis causes loss of bone strength and durability, and is the leading cause of bone fractures among the elderly. Osteoporosis is correctly regarded as problem that primarily affects older women. However, it is surprisingly widespread among older men, too. **More than five million men in the United States have osteoporosis,** according to the National Osteoporosis Foundation. Although it is eight times more common in women than in men, one in five men over the age of 65 will sustain bone fractures due to osteoporosis.

Osteoporosis develops less often in men than women because men have larger skeletons, because bone loss starts later and progresses more slowly, and because there is no rapid hormonal change in a man's life, such as menopause in a woman's life. Men are still at risk, however, especially from prolonged exposure to steroids or chronic disease, smoking and alcoholism, poor nutrition and bad exercise habits. Again, **early detection is the most important preventive measure,** and low adult bone density can be detected by plain radiographs (x-ray), ultrasound, and x-ray densitometry.

THE TOP 4 WAYS TO FIGHT OSTEOPOROSIS

- Eat foods or drink liquids high in calcium and vitamin D, both found in dairy products. Skim and 1% milk will provide these elements without adding animal fats to your diet.

- Moderate, regular weight-bearing exercise several times a week can have a dramatic result in fighting osteoporosis. Try lifting exercises with light weights and back extension exercises such as reverse butterflies.

- Don't smoke.

- Avoid excessive amounts of caffeine or alcohol.

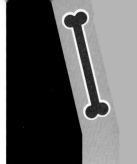

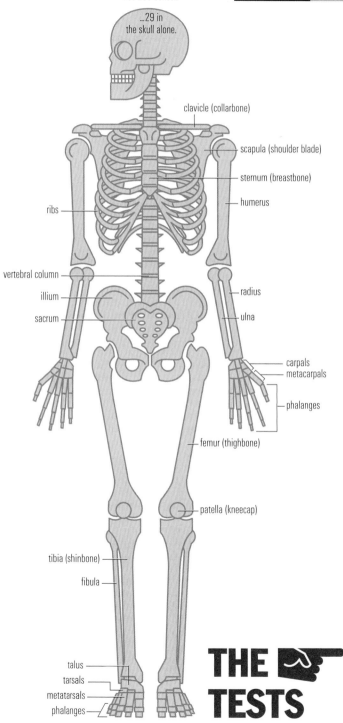

The average human adult has 206 bones...

...29 in the skull alone.

clavicle (collarbone)

scapula (shoulder blade)

sternum (breastbone)

humerus

ribs

vertebral column

illium

sacrum

radius

ulna

carpals

metacarpals

phalanges

femur (thighbone)

patella (kneecap)

tibia (shinbone)

fibula

talus

tarsals

metatarsals

phalanges

THE TESTS

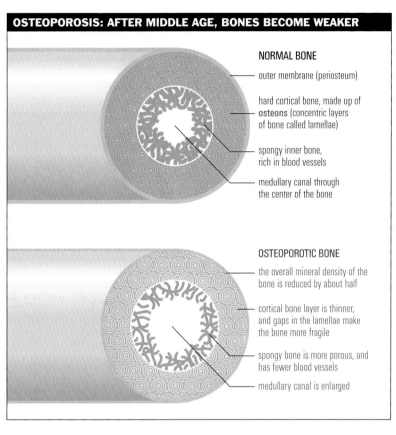

OSTEOPOROSIS: AFTER MIDDLE AGE, BONES BECOME WEAKER

NORMAL BONE

- outer membrane (periosteum)
- hard cortical bone, made up of osteons (concentric layers of bone called lamellae)
- spongy inner bone, rich in blood vessels
- medullary canal through the center of the bone

OSTEOPOROTIC BONE

- the overall mineral density of the bone is reduced by about half
- cortical bone layer is thinner, and gaps in the lamellae make the bone more fragile
- spongy bone is more porous, and has fewer blood vessels
- medullary canal is enlarged

Bone Densitometry

This is a safe and painless technique which utilizes x-rays to measure the absorption of photon radiation to determine bone density.

Procedure:

Different bones in the body are tested for density with photon radiation.

Results:

The images are used to determine bone mass, which is compared to standard mass for the patient's age, weight and gender. This test is used to screen and diagnose osteoporosis.

X-ray and Magnetic Resonance Imaging Tests

These generic tests (*described in Medical Terms at the end of this book*) are frequently used to diagnose fractures of bones and arthritis.

Blood Test for Calcium

Calcium is the most common mineral in the human body. It helps muscles contract, the heart beat, blood clotting and nerve impulses. This test examines the amount of calcium in the blood.

Procedure

Blood is drawn from a vein and sent to a lab for analysis.

Results

Too much calcium in the blood may indicate that calcium is being lost from bones. This may be an indication of hormone imbalance, cancer, or of kidney problems (see phosphorus, magnesium in Kidney chapter). There are two causes for calcium loss from bones: leaching and poor absorption from the gastrointestinal system (thyroid-related).

ALL ABOUT THE SPINE

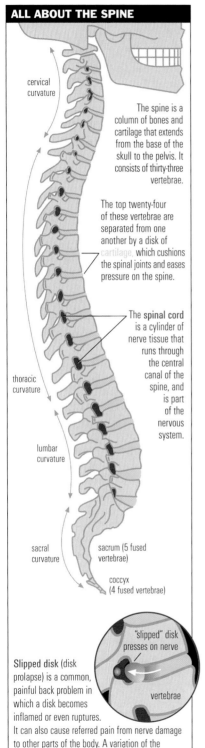

cervical
curvature

The spine is a column of bones and cartilage that extends from the base of the skull to the pelvis. It consists of thirty-three vertebrae.

The top twenty-four of these vertebrae are separated from one another by a disk of cartilage, which cushions the spinal joints and eases pressure on the spine.

The **spinal cord** is a cylinder of nerve tissue that runs through the central canal of the spine, and is part of the nervous system.

thoracic
curvature

lumbar
curvature

sacral
curvature

sacrum (5 fused vertebrae)

coccyx
(4 fused vertebrae)

"slipped" disk presses on nerve

vertebrae

Slipped disk (disk prolapse) is a common, painful back problem in which a disk becomes inflamed or even ruptures. It can also cause referred pain from nerve damage to other parts of the body. A variation of the myelogram, the diskogram, injects dye into the disk itself, and x-rays taken may show disk prolapse.

Bone Marrow Aspiration

The core of the bone, called the bone marrow, is where blood cells are manufactured. This procedure, in which a small portion of the bone is removed for analysis, is helpful in the diagnosis of leukemia and other varieties of cancer.

Procedure

Marrow may be extracted from the hip bone or from the breast bone. The skin in the area is cleaned and sterilized, and a local anaesthetic is injected into both the skin and bone area. A long hollow needle is then inserted through the skin and into the bone itself, puncturing it. The bone marrow layer is reached, and bone marrow is extracted and analyzed. Despite the anaesthetic, this test may be painful. After the procedure the patient may be bruised and tender.

Results

The marrow is tested for the types and numbers of red and white blood cells to determine the presence of anemia and other blood diseases, such as leukemia and cancer. The ability of the marrow to create new blood cells can be determined as well. The marrow can be cultured or even cloned for future use.

Nuclear Bone Scan

Because some areas of abnormal bone do not show up well on x-rays, a nuclear scan may be ordered to detect bone disease earlier and to better differentiate between normal and abnormal bone formation.

Procedure

After a radioactive substance (usually technetium TC-99) is injected into a vein, the patient must wait approximately 3 hours for the material to be absorbed into the bones. Diseased bone will absorb radioactivity differently than normal bone. The patient

more tests ☞

lies still on a table for up to an hour as the nuclear camera takes pictures. They may be taken of the entire skeleton, or of a certain part of the body.

Results

The camera converts the images into a picture which looks like a skeleton. Abnormal areas, indicating weak, decayed, or cancerous bone, will show up as "hot spots" on the pictures. Bone scans also provide valuable information for those with unexplained bone pain, and may reveal otherwise undetected fractures and infections.

Myelogram

For this specialized x-ray, dye is injected into the spinal canal (the cerebrospinal fluid that surrounds the spine) to detect abnormalities in the spinal cord and vertebrae.

BONE FACTS

Bones are not merely structural; bone is made up of calcium and phosphorus.

Hormones control growth and maintenance of bone tissue in the body.

Bones produce blood cells, formed in bone marrow, and act as storage sites for minerals in the body.

Bones need nutrition from the body throughout life.

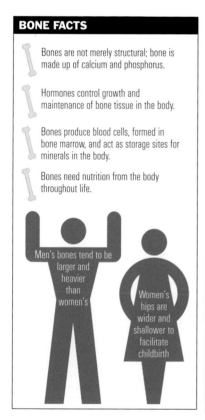

Men's bones tend to be larger and heavier than women's

Women's hips are wider and shallower to facilitate childbirth

Procedure

The patient must lie face down on an x-ray table. A local anesthetic is put into the back with a needle. A larger needle is inserted into the space between the vertebrae, and into the spinal canal, which contains cerebrospinal fluid (see also Spinal Tap), and a small amount of dye is injected. With the needle still in place, the patient and the table may be tilted to allow the dye to spread throughout the spinal cord. After x-rays are taken, the needle usually removes the dye (depending upon the type of dye used). Sometimes cerebrospinal fluid is removed for analysis as well.

Results

Numerous disorders can affect the spine and spinal cord, including degeneration and rupture of disks, infections in the spinal fluid, and arthritis of the vertebrae. The x-rays contribute to diagnosis of spinal cord abnormalities and tumors in the area as well.

This examination has potentially serious after-effects. The needle insertion, or spinal tap, may produce persistent leakage of cerebrospinal fluid, resulting in severe headache. The patient is often asked to remain in a reclining position for up to 12 hours after the test is concluded to avoid this problem. Depending on the material introduced, the patient may be at risk for seizures after the test.

Vitamin D Blood Test

Vitamin D is essential to the body because it helps calcium be absorbed by the body into bone and other tissue. It is present in dairy products and most products heavy in animal fats.

Procedure

Blood is drawn from a vein and sent to a lab for analysis.

20 minutes in the sun converts chemicals in the body into the recommended daily allowance of Vitamin D.

Results

A deficiency in the blood may point to a nutritional deficiency which weakens the skeleton, and may cause weak bones, called osteomalacia (the adult form of rickets). This is treated with vitamin D and calcium supplements.

For further information

National Institutes of Health Osteoporosis and Related Bone Diseases National Resource Center
1232 22nd Street NW
Washington, DC 20036-4603
(202) 223-0344 or 1(800) 624-BONE

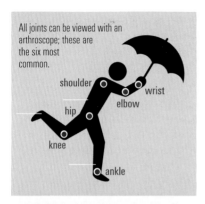

All joints can be viewed with an arthroscope; these are the six most common.

shoulder
wrist
elbow
hip
knee
ankle

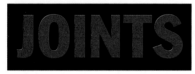

JOINTS

Joints are defined as the junction of two or more bones. They contain ligaments, tissue which connects bones; tendons, tissue which connects muscle to bone; cartilage, tissue which protects bones from rubbing each other directly; and membranes which line the entire joint surface. Joint problems include diseases such as arthritis, as well as malfunctions due to inflammation and injury. Specialists in arthritis and other afflictions of the joints are called rheumatologists.

Arthritis is not a single disorder, but the name of a collection of joint diseases which have a number of causes.

Osteoarthritis, or degenerative joint disease, is the most common form. It affects more than 21 million Americans, and is a leading cause of disability in the US. **Osteoarthritis** causes pain, swelling, creaking, and stiffness in one or more joints. Although almost 70% of those over age 70 have x-ray evidence of the disease, only half of these people suffer from pain or impaired mobility. Men are generally affected at an older age than women. Osteoarthritis can be treated with drugs, physical modalities, and fluids injected into joints to lubricate them. Septic arthritis results from direct infection of a joint with bacteria.

Rheumatoid arthritis, an auto-immune disorder, is one of the most severe forms of arthritis. The onset most frequently occurs in young to middle adulthood, but may occur at any age, even in childhood. It is a disease which causes the immune system to attack the body's own tissues. The joints of the fingers, wrists, toes, or other areas become swollen, painful, stiff —and in severe cases, deformed. Men are less vulnerable to rheumatoid arthritis than women.

In addition to arthritis, other common joint disorders include tears of joint tissue, such as the rotator cuff or other tendons. Tears or breaks can leave loose particles of cartilage in the joint as well, which can cause irritation.

Numbness, tingling or shooting pains in the hand and arm can be signs of **carpal tunnel syndrome** (median neuropathy, repetitive motion disorder). Anything that causes compression of the median nerve within the wrist can result in carpal tunnel syndrome. Common causes include overuse of the hand and wrist, swelling from arthritis, thyroid imbalance and diabetes.

Although the majority of patients complaining of carpal tunnel syndrome are women, men with repetitive motion jobs or continuous computer use are at risk, too. It may be treated with a stiff brace, worn at night to immobilize the wrist, steroids or corrective surgery.

Important advances in the diagnosis and treatment of joints, bones, ligaments, tendons, muscles, and nerves have led to a newly developed branch of orthopedics called sports medicine. Athletes, both amateur and professional, whose injuries might have been devastating only a few decades ago, are now examined and successfully treated with arthroscopy and quickly returned to the playing fields.

THE TOP 6 CONDITIONS ASSOCIATED WITH CARPAL TUNNEL SYNDROME

- Repetitive and forceful grasping of the hands.
- Repetitive bending of the wrists.
- Broken or dislocated wrist bones.
- Arthritis, especially rheumatoid arthritis.
- Thyroid imbalance.
- Diabetes.

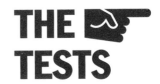

THE TESTS

INSIDE THE KNEE

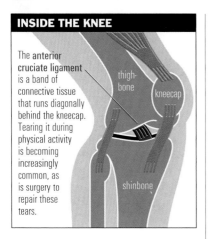

The anterior cruciate ligament is a band of connective tissue that runs diagonally behind the kneecap. Tearing it during physical activity is becoming increasingly common, as is surgery to repair these tears.

thigh-bone

kneecap

shinbone

Arthroscopy

In this test a specialized arthroscope allows the physician to see directly inside the joint, including all the bones and connective tissue.

Procedure

A local anesthetic is injected into the joint to be examined. Depending on the joint, a general anesthetic may be administered as well. A buttonhole-sized incision is made in the skin, and the arthroscope is inserted through the hole into the joint area. The doctor then uses the scope to examine the joint visually. Arthroscopy may be accompanied by arthroscopic surgery. Specialized surgical tools designed to repair torn tissue or remove fluid or loose fragments may be inserted through the same hole as the arthroscope. This type of surgery is preferable to an open surgical procedure (arthrotomy) because of its precision and because it opens up only a small hole in the skin.

Because of the use of anesthesia, patients will be asked to refrain from food or water after midnight the day before the arthroscopy is performed.

Results

This test allows the doctor to see the bones in a joint, the tissues connecting them, and their functions can be directly viewed. The patient may experience discomfort and swelling

after the test is completed and should limit physical activity for several days. Physicians generally recommend that the patient not drive after the test.

Arthrocentesis (Joint Aspiration)

Synovial fluid lubricates the joints of the body. If a joint is painful or swollen, the doctor may perform an arthrocentesis to remove excessive synovial fluid or to examine the fluid.

Procedure

After the skin over the joint is cleaned and sterilized, a local anesthetic is injected. The doctor then inserts a needle into the joint cavity to withdraw synovial fluid. Despite the anaesthetic, patients may experience mild discomfort when the needle is inserted.

Results

Depending upon the reason for the arthrocentesis, the synovial fluid may be examined after removal. The synovial fluid white blood count is a good indicator for inflammation. Other studies that may be ordered include analysis of uric acid crystals (if gout is suspected) or microscopic examination for bacteria and cultures (if infection is suspected).

Arthrogram

Regular x-rays of joints have limited ability to differentiate between types of joint tissue. In this test dye is injected into the joints, which makes it possible to distinguish the soft tissue structures within the joints. It is most often performed on the knee.

Procedure

The joint to be examined is cleaned and sterilized. A needle is inserted into the joint, and dye is injected. X-rays are taken of the joint from different angles. The patient moves the joint around so that the dye distributes itself well.

HIP REPLACEMENT

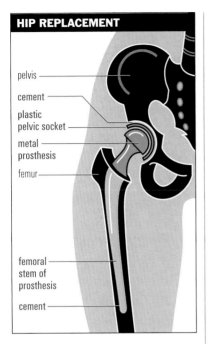

pelvis

cement

plastic
pelvic socket

metal
prosthesis

femur

femoral
stem of
prosthesis

cement

Results

These x-rays can show the status of soft tissue in the joint. They can show tears and loose pieces of tissue or bone, as well as the functioning of the joint. Arthroscopy is usually more accurate than an arthrogram and is often preferred to this test.

Uric Acid Blood Test

Gout is the painful swelling of the joints due to excessive accumulation of uric acid. Gout can occur as a hereditary, metabolic condition, or may be due to kidney malfunction. The body can fail to excrete enough uric acid.

Procedure

Blood is drawn from a vein and sent to a lab for analysis.

Results

Elevated uric acid levels predisposes patients to attacks of gout. Kidney diseases may result in elevated uric acid levels. Conversely, long standing elevation of uric acid can result in kidney damage.

For this test, see **BRAIN** *page 23*

Magnetic Resonance Imaging (MRI)

Used to diagnose joint problems, especially in the knee and shoulder.

Erythrocyte Sedimentation Rate (ESR Blood Test)

When blood is withdrawn and allowed to stand in a special tube, red blood cells settle at varying rates. This test measures how quickly blood settles. An increased rate of settling often is a good indicator of the presence of inflammatory conditions (e.g. arthritis), while a slow or normal rate is usually present in healthy individuals.

Procedure

Blood is drawn from a vein and sent to a lab for analysis.

Results

This test measures how much a sample of red blood cells settle in an hour, aiding in diagnosis of diseases such as arthritis and cancer. Inflammatory and other diseases, as well as pregnancy, will promote faster settling.

Tennis elbow occurs because of overuse or weakness in the muscles attached to the elbow, which move the wrist and fingers. The pain is aggravated by heavy lifting, racquet sports, and gardening. Steroids, ice, painkillers and rest are possible treatments.

For further information

National Institute of Arthritis and Musculoskeletal & Skin Diseases Information Clearinghouse
National Institute of Health (NIH)
1 AMS Circle
Bethesda, MD 20892-3675
(301) 495-4484
www.nih.gov/niams

The Arthritis Foundation
www.arthritis.org

American Fibromyalgia Syndrome Assoc.
www.afsafund.org

BLOOD

There are more tests of blood than there are of any other body component, and **blood testing reveals much more information about the body than just blood disorders.** Hematology is the name given to the discipline or specialty that studies and treats disorders of the blood.

The main function of blood is as a transport system, carrying oxygen and nutrients to all organs and tissues of the body. It is a river that travels through 60,000 miles of veins and arteries. Blood also has a major role in fighting infections.

About half of blood is made up of red blood cells, white blood cells, and platelets, most of which are made in bone marrow. Red blood cells, about 40% of blood, are containers for the protein called hemoglobin. Hemoglobin takes oxygen from the lungs and carries it to the rest of the body, and carries carbon dioxide back to the lungs for expulsion from the body. White blood cells are part of the immune system, designed to fight viruses, bacteria, fungi and parasites. Platelets are part of the blood's own maintenance system, helping blood clot and repair broken blood vessels. White blood cells and platelets together make up less than 5% of blood.

The rest of blood consists of a liquid called plasma. Plasma contains dissolved minerals, proteins, sugars and fats, which are transported to organs and tissues to sustain those body parts. As tissues use these nutrients, they also produce waste, which the blood takes to the kidneys for elimination from the body. The liver also processes some waste products, excreting bile. Hormones also travel through the blood, giving instructions to various organs.

THE 3 TYPES OF BLOOD TEST

- **Hematological tests** involve looking at the components of the blood itself.

- **Biochemical tests** look at chemicals in the blood, which sometimes indicate organ malfunction.

- **Microbiological tests** examine the blood for bacteria, viruses and other small organisms and many measure the body's defense against them.

Almost all blood tests begin by drawing blood from the patient through a hypodermic needle (a procedure called venipuncture). Once a quantity of blood has been drawn, it can be tested for evidence of an almost endless number of hormones, bacteria, antibodies, proteins, minerals, and otherwise normal ingredients such as hemoglobin and platelets. Since the levels of many chemicals in the blood fluctuate during the day, blood is often drawn early in the morning, before the body has processed any nutrients (i.e. breakfast). **Because the blood can change from day to day, it is not uncommon for repeat testing to be ordered.** Blood tests are often done to monitor a chemical in the blood over time as well, especially to see how the body reacts to a new drug. For example, cholesterol levels are checked to monitor the effect of a lipid lowering drug.

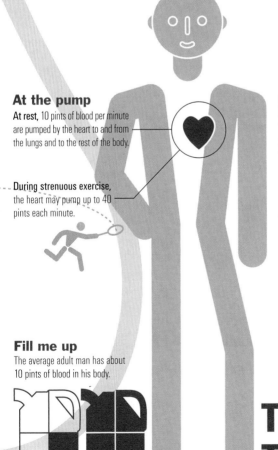

At the pump
At rest, 10 pints of blood per minute are pumped by the heart to and from the lungs and to the rest of the body.

During strenuous exercise, the heart may pump up to 40 pints each minute.

Check your blood cells, sir?
The body must produce 2,400,000 new red blood cells every second to maintain normal blood.

One cubic millimeter of blood (*that's about this much:* ■) usually contains between 4 and 5 million red blood cells. The average person has about 35 trillion red blood cells, which have a lifespan of approximately 120 days. Blood removed for transfusion is only good for about 20 days.

Fill me up
The average adult man has about 10 pints of blood in his body.

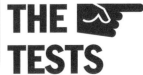

THE
TESTS

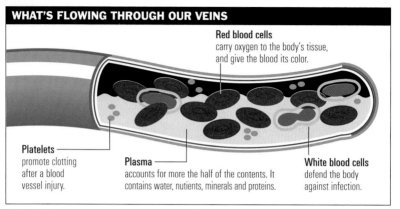

WHAT'S FLOWING THROUGH OUR VEINS

Red blood cells
carry oxygen to the body's tissue, and give the blood its color.

Platelets
promote clotting after a blood vessel injury.

Plasma
accounts for more the half of the contents. It contains water, nutients, minerals and proteins.

White blood cells
defend the body against infection.

Blood Pressure

Blood pressure is the pressure or tension of the blood against the artery walls. It increases with physical activity and decreases with sleep.

Procedure

An instrument called a sphygmomanometer is used to take blood pressure. A cuff is wrapped around the arm of the patient, and the doctor, nurse or technician pumps the cuff full of air, obstructing circulation in the arm. A stethoscope is placed over the artery in the arm. The cuff is then loosened, and as circulation resumes, the pressure is noted. The pressure is noted again as the sound of the blood against the artery markedly diminishes and then disappears.

Results

Blood pressure readings are conventionally given as a fraction. The top number, called systolic pressure, refers to the pressure right after the heart has contracted, at its peak. The bottom number, diastolic pressure, measures pressure when the heart is relaxed. 120/80 is given as a "normal" figure, but blood pressure is relative to each individual. Older patients are considered within normal range up to 140/90. High blood pressure can cause blood vessels to weaken or burst, and is a factor in heart attacks, heart failure and strokes. High blood pressure also contributes to generalized arteriosclerosis or hardening of the arteries, and the development of kidney failure.

> Over 58 million Americans have high blood pressure, often showing no visible symptoms. High blood pressure and blockages of arteries are also connected.

Venography (Phlebography)

Blood clots most commonly occur in the veins of the legs. These clots can lead to poor circulation. If dislodged, they can travel to the lung, causing serious damage or death. This specialized angiogram specifically looks for clots in the veins of the legs.

Procedure

The patient must not eat for several hours before the test. The skin of the leg to be examined is sterilized, and a dye is injected into a vein at the top of the foot. Through either tourniquets or gravity, the dye spreads throughout the leg, and x-rays are taken. Sometimes an examination table that tilts is used.

Results

The x-rays of the leg will show how blood flows through them. Clots in the body will stop or impede the dye from traveling further and show up clearly on the x-rays. These can then be treated with blood thinners or surgery.

Anemia is a condition in which there is not enough hemoglobin in the bloodstream. Iron deficiency is a frequent cause. Anemia prevents adequate oxygen transportation in the body, and can be quite serious. Heart and brain function can be impaired by not enough oxygen, and muscles can tire very easily. There are several types of anemia. One which can be tested for is sickle cell anemia, a genetic disease, which causes red blood cells to deform and clog blood vessels.

Complete Blood Count (CBC), Red Blood Cell or White Blood Cell

This is the most frequent blood test performed. It contains many tests which examine the health and make-up of the blood, providing general, broad diagnostic information.

Procedure

Blood is drawn from a vein and sent to a lab for analysis by machine.

Results

The test counts and analyzes red blood cells, hemoglobin levels, the hematocrit (a measure of how much of total blood is made up of red blood cells), white blood cells, and platelets. Too few red blood cells and a low hematocrit mean anemia is present and a search for possible causes, such as infection, iron deficiency, internal bleeding and cancer should be undertaken. Further blood tests which measure red blood cell size are often done to help determine the type of anemia.

A high white cell count indicates infection, inflammation and, occasionally, the presence of cancer. Analysis of white blood cells can also reveal the cause of infection or suggest leukemia or other blood diseases. A lack of platelets can affect the clotting ability of the blood, or can be a sign of leukemia. Usually a smear analysis is performed as well, allowing blood cells to be examined under a microscope.

Blood Typing

Blood type is determined by the presence (or absence) of certain proteins on the surface of the red blood cell. Laboratories commonly test for two "systems" of such proteins: ABO (A,B, or no ABO protein) and Rh (positive or negative). The presence or absence of components of either system determines the exact blood type of an individual. This test is done before most surgical procedures and transfusions to determine the patient's blood type and to help prevent serious reactions.

Procedure

Blood is drawn from a vein and sent to a lab for analysis.

Results

There are a total of eight major blood types: A, B, AB, and O, each Rh positive or negative.

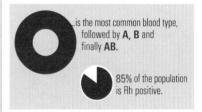

...is the most common blood type, followed by **A, B** and finally **AB**.

85% of the population is Rh positive.

Alcohol

Alcohol is normally not found in the body. The most common way it gets there is through consumption of alcoholic beverages. While most often used by police to detect drunken driving, it is sometimes tested for in hospitals if coma or abnormal behavior is present.

Procedure

Blood is drawn from a vein and sent to a lab for analysis.

more tests ☞

Results

The test shows alcohol as a percentage of blood content. Anything over 0.05% impairs normal hand-eye coordination. Most states now have drunk driving laws which define inebriation between 0.08 and 0.10%. By 2004, a state must use 0.08% as the standard in order to continue receiving federal highway funds.

For these tests, see **LUNGS** *pages 52-57*

Arterial Blood Gases
Carboxyhemoglobin

Blood Culture or Wound Culture

If infection is found in the blood, it can be very serious, because it indicates that the problem may spread through the body to multiple sites, potentially causing organ malfunction or failure, and shock. If a fever develops with no cause, this test is often ordered.

Procedure

Blood is drawn or pus is obtained and sent to a lab for analysis.

Results

The sample is cultured in a lab, and if any growth results, it indicates an infection. This can be treated with antibiotics or by other measures.

Blood Albumin and Globulin

The presence of these proteins in plasma can be indicative of specific kinds of disease, as well as an individual's nutritional status.

Procedure

Blood is drawn from a vein and sent to a lab for analysis.

Results

Too much globulin in the blood is found in patients with certain kinds of inflammatory (e.g. autoimmune) diseases, as well as some forms of cancer. Too little albumin is often due to kidney disease, various other chronic illnesses, and poor nutrition.

White blood cells which attack bacteria have a lifespan of only 6 to 9 hours. The exception is lymphocytes, which are made in lymph glands, not in bone marrow, and can last up to 10 years in the bloodstream. Some lymphocytes (type B) are made in the bone marrow. Lymphocytes form antibodies and are key disease fighters. They are the part of the blood which the AIDS virus attacks.

Coombs' Test

This procedure tests for antibodies which attack the patient's own red blood cells.

Procedure

Blood is drawn from a vein and sent to a lab for analysis.

Results

Some antibodies are in the blood naturally and attack foreign substances in the body. If an incompatible blood transfusion has been performed, or in certain types of anemia, however, antibodies will attack healthy blood cells in the body. The Coombs' test will detect these antibodies.

For this test, see **JOINTS** *pages 104-107*

Erythrocyte Sedimentation Rate (ESR, sed rate)

Infectious Disease Antibody

Almost any kind of infection makes the body produce specific antibodies, which may help to combat the disease. Many of these antibodies can be measured and used to diagnose illness.

Procedure

Blood is drawn from a vein and sent

to a lab for analysis.

Results

Each test measures levels of antibodies (titers) to a specific infection or prior vaccination for that infection. The rubella antibody test, for example, measures antibody titers to German measles. This test is often given before marriage because infection with German measles can cause birth defects.

NORMAL & VARICOSE VEINS

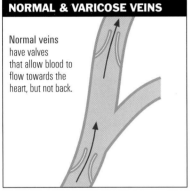

Normal veins have valves that allow blood to flow towards the heart, but not back.

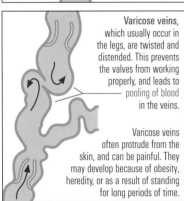

Varicose veins, which usually occur in the legs, are twisted and distended. This prevents the valves from working properly, and leads to pooling of blood in the veins.

Varicose veins often protrude from the skin, and can be painful. They may develop because of obesity, heredity, or as a result of standing for long periods of time.

For these tests see **HEART** *pages 44-51*

Lipids/Cholesterol, Triglycerides, HDL, LDL

Apolipoproteins

Heart Enzyme, CPK, CK, SGOT, or LDH

Vitamin B1

Hematocrit

Antimyocardial Antibodies

Iron, TIBC, Ferratin

Iron is extremely important for the body because it is necessary for hemoglobin production. Iron is used and stored in the bone marrow. These tests are commonly used to diagnose such conditions as anemia (is iron deficiency the cause?) and iron overload (a condition called hemochromatosis).

Procedure

Blood is drawn from a vein and sent to a lab for analysis.

Results

Iron can be tested for directly, but this test can be misleading. TIBC measures the amount of proteins in the blood to which iron binds for transport. The ferratin test measures the amount of iron in the form in which it is stored in the body. All three tests are looking for low or high levels of iron. Iron-deficiency anemia is the most common diagnosis from this test.

> Iron-deficiency anemia arises from three causes: Low levels of iron in the diet; chronic blood loss, usually from intestinal bleeding disorders, or inadequate absorption of iron from the intestinal tract.

For this test, see **BRAIN** *pages 18-25*

Hormone Testing

Lead

Animals naturally have no lead in their body whatsoever. Because of use of lead and lead-based products in modern society (particularly in lead-based paint), however, lead has been introduced into our bodies as well. High levels of lead can be quite toxic.

Procedure

Blood is drawn from a vein and sent to a lab for analysis.

Results

Blood will reveal elevated levels of lead, if present. X-rays can also reveal lead deposits in bones. Because the body excretes lead very slowly, chelating or binding agents may be prescribed to help eliminate it faster.

Acute lead poisoning, the rapid intake of a lot of lead, is rare but can be fatal. Babies and toddlers are at highest risk for chronic lead poisoning, mostly through eating old paint that has peeled off walls. Children and adults both may be exposed to elevated levels of lead through consumption of acidic food or drink (orange juice, tomato sauce) that has been stored or cooked in lead-glazed or lead-soldered containers (often brought home from overseas as souvenirs). Adults who work in manufacturing plants which use lead are also at risk.

Buildup of lead can have many effects, including brain, nerve, and red blood cell damage. Toxic levels of lead in the body can also cause mental impairment, especially in children. Lead accumulates primarily in the bones and may be released by osteoporosis.

Prothrombin Time, Partial Thromboplastin Time, Bleeding Time

Blood clotting is extremely important to survival. If blood never clotted, wounds would bleed indefinitely. Surgery would be impossible. Proteins in the blood work with platelets to promote clotting in normal people, but some lack sufficient quantities of the necessary agents. These tests are used to see how well blood clots, and are given before some surgical procedures.

Procedure

Blood is drawn from a vein and sent to a lab for analysis.

Results

The prothrombin time and partial prothombin time tests measure the amount of clotting substances in the blood to make sure that blood will clot normally during and after an operation. The bleeding time test makes sure the platelets are present and functioning properly.

If blood takes too long to clot, it may be an indicator of liver disease or an inherited clotting disorder. For patients who are taking prescription anticoagulants such as coumadin (warfarin) to prevent dangerous clots from travelling to vital organs, the clotting time is slower. Prothrombin time tests are routinely ordered to ensure that clotting time is neither too fast nor too slow.

Reticulocyte Count

Reticulocytes are immature red blood cells just released by the bone marrow. Over several days, they grow into mature red blood cells.

Procedure

Blood is drawn from a vein and sent to a lab for analysis.

Results

This test measures the ability of bone marrow to produce red blood cells. It also assists in the detection of some types of anemia and measures the effectiveness of certain vitamins and minerals (e.g., iron and folic acid) to stimulate red blood cell production. Low reticulocyte counts generally indicate a failure of the bone marrow to respond normally (e.g., iron deficiency, blood diseases such as leukemia and cancer).

For these tests, see **LIVER**, *pp. 58-65*

Mono Spot Blood Test

Alanine Aminotransferase (ALT) or Serum Glutamic-Pyruvic Transminase Blood Test (SGPT)

Alpha-fetoprotein Blood Test (AFP)

Alkaline Phosphatase Blood Test (ALP)

Bilirubin Blood Test

Protein, Albumin, Serum Protein, Globulin, and Serum Electrophoresis Blood Tests

Hepatitis Blood Test

For these tests, see **KIDNEYS** *pages 66-73*

Electrolytes

Magnesium

Osmolality

Phosphorus

Sodium

Blood Urea Nitrogen (BUN), Creatinine, Creatinine Clearance

Renal Assay, Plasma

For these tests, see **GALLBLADDER & PANCREAS** *pages 74-79*

Amylase

C-peptide

Glucose

Hemoglobin A1C (Glycohemoglobin)

Ketones

Lipase

For this test, see **UPPER GI** *pages 80-85*

Gastrin

For this test, see **LOWER GI** *pages 86-91*

Carcinoembryonic Antigen (CEA)

For the following tests, see **REPRODUCTIVE SYSTEM** *pages 92-97*

Prostate Specific Antigen (PSA)

AIDS Blood Serology

Gonorrhea or Chlamydia Blood Test

Syphilis Blood Test

For this test, see **BONES** *pages 98-103*

Vitamin D

For this test, see **JOINTS** *pages 104-107*

Uric Acid Blood Test

Angiography (Angiogram), Magnetic Resonance Imaging (MRI), and Ultrasound (Ultrasonography)

These valuable procedures for observing many aspects of organs and systems throughout the body are frequently utilized to analyze aspects of the vascular system. They may be used for both diagnosis and monitoring. (*See Medical Terms at the back of this book for descriptions of these procedures.*)

For Further Information

The American Society of Hematology
1200 19th Street NW #300
Washington, DC 20036
202- 857-1118
www.hematology.org

National Heart, Lung, and Blood Institute
9000 Rockville Pike
Bethesda, MD 20892
1-301-496-4236
www.nhlbi.nih.gov/

BloodLine - The Online Resource for Hematology Education and News
www.bloodline.net

Why Do You Need A Laboratory Test?
www.pscls.org/lab_test.html

Anesthesia

Anesthesia refers to any of a number of chemicals given to a patient to take some of the discomfort and pain out of medical procedures. There are two types of anesthesia, general and local. A general anesthetic makes the patient unconscious for a given amount of time. It is usually administered by an anesthesiologist before many types of invasive surgery, but rarely for medical tests. The chemical can be given in a gas form through a mask, or injected into a vein. A local anesthetic is usually a numbing agent which kills pain in one part of the body, but the patient remains awake. This is commonly used before invasive diagnostic tests. It comes in solution form, which can be sprayed or rubbed on (frequently used in the mouth and throat) or can be injected, usually near the site of the test.

Angiogram

An angiogram is an x-ray of a blood vessel, usually with a radio opaque dye injected into the area to be photographed, making certain parts of the picture stand out more clearly. Air-filled organs do not show up on x-rays, so these are often targets of the dyes used. The material is called radio opaque, because it appears opaque or white on x-rays. The test is used to study a particular blood vessel or group of blood vessels. If blood vessels are blocked and the contrast medium cannot pass through, this becomes evident. During a typical procedure, a patient is injected with the contrast material, which is allowed to spread through the blood vessels. A fluoroscope is used to watch it spread, which is an x-ray scanner which projects a moving picture of the body onto a TV screen. Unlike x-rays, it is not a still image. Once the dye is in place, still x-rays are taken. The dye often causes a flushed or faint feeling and causes an allergic reaction in some people. The patient should disclose all allergies before the test is done. The contrast material, combined with the x-rays, expose the body to amounts of radiation that are too small to be considered a risk.

Biopsy

Biopsy refers to the removal of tissue from a living body to study it. There are two types of biopsy, excision and aspiration. Excision biopsy refers to the removal of tissue invasively, with a scalpel or similar tool. For example, a surgeon may open up the skin of the breast and withdraw a piece of tissue to test it for cancer. An aspiration biopsy is usually performed with a needle, which is inserted through the skin into the area being investigated. Cells are then drawn up through the needle into a syringe and sent for analysis. This can also be performed on the breast, and is in fact the preferred method of testing there. The cells in either test can be cultured for bacteria or other infections, examined for cancer, and tested for genetic make-up. Cancerous cells can be tested for malignancy. Sometimes an ultrasound or fluoroscopy (see x-ray) is performed to guide the exact location of the biopsy. See also endoscopy, which sometimes involves biopsy procedures.

Catheter

The catheter is a flexible tube that can be inserted into the body for a number of reasons. The most common is to act as a drain when the function of an organ may be impaired by medication, surgery or disease. A urinary catheter is inserted up into the urethra into the bladder. Catheters can also be inserted into the bloodstream through a vein. In this case they are used to pump in and withdraw different fluids. The primary risk of catheterization is that the introduction of the catheter may dislodge buildup on the walls of a vein and send a clot towards the heart, where it could cause a heart attack. In the bladder, a catheter could puncture the urethra or bladder, but this is unlikely.

CAT or CT Scan

Traditional x-rays use the human body to cast a "shadow" onto x-ray film. In Computerized Axial Tomography, or CT scan, however, a scanner measures radiation as it bounces off different tissues and by combining these readings can give an accurate 3-D picture of the body to doctors. The scan displays cross-sectional slices of the body, accurately identifying tumors, blockages, and fluids   It actually uses less radiation than a traditional x-ray scan. CT scans have reduced the need for angiography and other tests in many cases, ensuring less risk and invasiveness for the patient. During this test, the patient lies on a table which slides into the scanner, a large, doughnut-shaped box. The scanner then shoots x-rays at the patient and measures the response. A sedative may be administered before the test, and if necessary, the patient may be given a laxative to clear the bowel of stool or gas. Rarely, a dye is injected, as in an angiogram. The only difficulty in the test lies in keeping perfectly still for the duration, sometimes up to an hour.

Endoscopy

Endoscopy simply refers to a test in which an examination device is passed into the body through an orifice or hole to examine its internal workings. The tube can be inserted into any orifice of the body, such as the mouth, nose, anus or urethra. With the aid of fiber optic technology, these tubes are now usually small and flexible, although rigid tubes are still used for some techniques. The endoscope, as the tube is called, can perform many functions once inserted into the body. The primary function is to give the doctor a picture of the organs being examined. A camera and light source are at the tip of every endoscope, and transmit pictures which appear on a television screen. Needles can be passed down the endoscope and used to inject or withdraw fluids for analysis. These fluids can be cultured for bacteria, or tested for blood or other components.

The endoscope also gives the doctor access to tissues for biopsy. Fluid can be extracted with a needle for a biopsy, or a small clamp can be passed through the endoscope to withdraw a piece of tissue. The endoscopy is much less invasive and painful than surgery, and only occasionally requires sedation or anesthesia.

Heart Attack

(myocardial infarction)
About one million people suffer from heart attacks every year in the US. One third of these attacks are fatal. A heart attack is the sudden death of a part of the heart muscle, which may cause the heart to have an abnormal rhythm or stop entirely. Sometimes the heart assumes an

abnormal rhythm when it begins to beat again, and its overall strength and structure can be weakened. A heart attack may cause severe, non-stop chest pain. Victims may be short of breath, become nauseated or lose consciousness. Heart attacks, however, may generate few symptoms at all. Heart attacks are caused by lack of blood to part of the heart muscle, usually because of clogged blood vessels.

Men have different symptoms than women; smokers are more likely to be at risk than non-smokers. Other risk factors include age, diet, stress and high blood pressure. Heart attacks are usually diagnosed with an EKG and blood tests.

Hypertension
(high blood pressure)
While blood pressure fluctuates with every individual, and stress or physical activity elevate blood pressure, a patient is said to have high blood pressure when the readings lie outside the normal range (140/90) at rest. Blood pressure increases with age. In most people with hypertension, there is no obvious cause, although diet and lifestyle issues, such as smoking, obesity and kidney disorders, put individuals at risk. Certain ethnic groups are more at risk for hypertension. Many cases of high blood pressure show no symptoms and are often not discovered until a physical examination. About 15 million people in the United States are being treated for high blood pressure. If untreated, it can lead to heart failure, stroke, or kidney damage. Prolonged high blood pressure leads to buildup in the arteries and a weakening of the heart. Changes in lifestyle, such as quitting smoking, drinking and eating fatty foods, are often recommended to combat hypertension, but drugs can be prescribed as well.

Magnetic Resonance Imaging (MRI)
This test puts the patient inside what is essentially a big magnet, which infuses sections of the body with a radio pulse. Different tissue densities and movements within the body respond differently to such magnetic pulses, and thus show up differently on the magnetic sensor. The patient lies down on a table which slides inside the doughnut-shaped magnet.

Today, both closed and open MRIs are available, the latter for large or claustrophobic patients. The table continues to move in small increments during the test, and the magnet makes a lot of noise as the pictures are taken. Like a CAT scan, slices of images are taken which can later be combined to make a detailed 3-D image. The test can detect tumors, abnormal blood flow, inflammations and muscle tears. The whole procedure can take from 30 to 90 minutes. Metal can disrupt the test, so anyone with a pacemaker or other piece of metal permanently installed in the body should not have the test. Fillings in teeth, which may buzz slightly during the test, are an exception. The test is safer than x-rays because there is no exposure to radiation or anything else deemed harmful.

Nuclear Scan
In this test, radioactive materials are attached to foods or chemicals that are normally found in the body. The choice of substance to which the

radioactive substance is attached depends on the organ being studied. Chemicals which are naturally used by the kidney, for example, will be utilized when the kidney is under observation. The radioactive foods or chemicals are either swallowed or injected, after which the patient waits until the material reaches the organ to be studied. Different types of tissue absorb the chemicals differently. This gives nuclear scans an advantage over x-rays: the function of an organ is more clearly visible, although the detail is not as great as that of x-rays. Nuclear or "gamma" cameras then take pictures of the organ to detect abnormalities. The gamma camera is somewhat like a Geiger counter, absorbing radiation patterns from the treated tissue. Abnormal bones and organs absorb material at different rates, and thus will show up differently on the scan. This can indicate cancer and infections. SPECT and PET scans are specialized nuclear scans which highlight tissues with metabolic rates higher than normal tissue. The radioactive materials pose no allergy risks, are low in radiation and move completely out of the body within a few days.

Stroke

A stroke occurs when blood supply to the brain is interrupted or when bleeding occurs, causing brain damage. Strokes are fatal in about one third of all cases, cause a significant disability in one third of all cases, and have no long-term ill effects in one third of cases. High blood pressure, or hypertension, is one big risk factor. Age is another. An older person is more prone to stroke, and men have them more often than women. Damage to one side of the brain will cause paralysis in the opposite side of the body. CT scans can be done to diagnose a stroke and also find its source, such as a blood clot.

Ultrasound

Unlike x-ray type scans, which take still pictures of a moment in time, ultrasound provides a moving picture of the interior of the body. High frequency sound waves are passed through the body using a transducer, a pen-like instrument. These waves bounce back to the transducer at different speeds, depending on how far they travel and on the density of the material they hit. The waves are interpreted by a computer and translated into a picture. This test can paint a picture of the organs of the body, their shape and function. Often done to locate an organ for biopsy, this test is considered completely safe and painless.

X-ray

The x-ray is a type of light wave that can pass through solid material. The less dense a material, the more transparent it is to x-rays. Transmitting x-rays through a body, then onto a piece of film yields a detailed picture of the tissues of varying densities. During routine x-rays, the patient stands or lies next to the x-ray camera. The photographic plate is then placed on the other side of the patient. When the "picture" is taken, x-rays are transmitted through the patient and onto the film. X-rays are not without risk, and although amount of radiation imparted to the body is usually very small the patient should be given a lead shield to place over the reproductive organs to block excess radiation.

120·ACKNOWLEDGEMENTS

Digby and **Kay Diehl** for their heroic efforts in research and writing.

Nigel Holmes of **Explanation Graphics** for his talent in making information come alive on a printed page.

Adam Graham Silverman for his assistance with much of the research.

Sharon Stea for her assistance in design and production.

The following distinguished members of the medical and scientific community have been most generous with their time, their knowledge, and their insights. To each, we say thank you.

DickAugspurger, M.D., Medical Director, **UnitedHealthcare of Colorado**

Richard A. Baker, M.D., Head of Radiology, **Lahey Clinic**, Burlington, MA

William A. Barnett, O.D., **South River Eye Care**, Edgewater, MD and **Bowie Optometric Group**, Bowie, MD

Paul D. Brant, O.D., Cambridge, MD

Jim Garfield, M.D., Medical Director, **UnitedHealthcare of Ohio**

Jonathon Garvas, M.D., Medical Director, **UnitedHealthcare of Florida**

Allen Grimes, M.D., Medical Director, **UnitedHealthcare of Kentucky**

Doug Hasbrouck, M.D., Medical Director, **UnitedHealthcare of Utah**

Mike Hawkins, M.D., Medical Director, **UnitedHealthcare of Texas**

Dick Justman, M.D., Medical Director, **UnitedHealthcare**, Mineapolis, MN

Tony Kazlauskas, M.D., Senior Medical Director, **UnitedHealthcare of New England**

Craig Keyes, M.D., Medical Director, **UnitedHealthcare of New York**

Rusty King, M.D., Medical Director, **UnitedHealthcare of Louisianna**

Julie Lindahl, M.D., Medical Director, **Golden Valley Care Management Center**, Golden Valley, MN

Bill Lynagh, M.D., Medical Director, **UnitedHealthcare of North Carolina**

John Mach, M.D., Chief Medical Officer, **Ovations**, a **UnitedHealth Group** company, Minneapolis, MN

David F. Miller, O.D., **TLC Laser Eye Center**, Annapolis, MD

Richard J. Raskin, M.D., Vice President and Chief Medical Director, **UnitedHealthcare of Ohio**

Michael Rosen, M.D., Medical Director, **UnitedHealthcare of Connecticut**

Robert S. Stutman, O.D., **Edward Wasloski, O.D.** and **Randall V. Wong, M.D.**, **Omni Eye Specialists**, Baltimore, MD

David Yalowitz, M.D., **UnitedHealthcare of Mid-Atlantic**